SCID-5-CV

STRUCTURED CLINICAL INTERVIEW FOR DSM-5® DISORDERS

CLINICIAN VERSION

Michael B. First, M.D.
Professor of Clinical Psychiatry, Columbia University, and Research Psychiatrist,
Division of Clinical Phenomenology, New York State Psychiatric Institute,
New York, New York

Janet B. W. Williams, Ph.D.
Professor Emerita of Clinical Psychiatric Social Work (in Psychiatry and in
Neurology), Columbia University, and Research Scientist and Deputy Chief,
Biometrics Research Department (Retired), New York State Psychiatric Institute,
New York, New York; and Senior Vice President of Global Science,
MedAvante, Inc., Hamilton, New Jersey

Rhonda S. Karg, Ph.D.
Research Psychologist, Division of Behavioral Health and
Criminal Justice Research, RTI International, Durham, North Carolina

Robert L. Spitzer, M.D.
Professor Emeritus of Psychiatry, Columbia University, and
Research Scientist and Chief, Biometrics Research Department (Retired),
New York State Psychiatric Institute, New York, New York

Patient: _____

Clinician: _____

Date of
Interview: _____ _____ _____
           month   day   year

Contents

List of Abbreviations

ADHD	Attention-Deficit/Hyperactivity Disorder
AMC	Another Medical Condition
GAD	Generalized Anxiety Disorder
GMC	General Medical Condition
(I)	Intoxication
(I/W)	Intoxication/Withdrawal
OC	Obsessive-Compulsive
OCD	Obsessive-Compulsive Disorder
PTSD	Posttraumatic Stress Disorder
(W)	Withdrawal

"**Note**" in boldface reflects the inclusion of notes as contained in the DSM-5 criteria.

"*NOTE*" in italics and all-capital letters indicates specific guidance or instructions for rating the criteria or conducting the SCID-5-CV interview.

SCID-5-CV DIAGNOSTIC SUMMARY SCORE SHEET

Schizophrenia Spectrum and Other Psychotic Disorders

Current	Past History	Disorder		
		Schizophrenia (p. 44/**C25**)		
☐	☐	F20.9		
		Schizophreniform Disorder (p. 44/**C26**)		
☐	☐	F20.81		
		Schizoaffective Disorder (p. 44/**C27**)		
☐	☐	F25.0	Bipolar Type	
☐	☐	F25.1	Depressive Type	
		Delusional Disorder (p. 44/**C28**)		
☐	☐	F22		
		Brief Psychotic Disorder (p. 44/**C29**)		
☐	☐	F23		

	Lifetime	
		Psychotic Disorder Due to Another Medical Condition (p. 38/**C6**, p. 39/**C8**, p. 40/**C12**, p. 41/**C17**, p. 42/**C21**, p. 43/**C24**)
	☐	F06.2 With Delusions
	☐	F06.0 With Hallucinations
		Substance/Medication-Induced Psychotic Disorder (p. 38/**C6**, p. 39/**C8**, p. 40/**C12**, p. 41/**C17**, p. 42/**C21**, p. 43/**C24**)
	☐	F___.___[1] Indicate specific substance and diagnostic code: _____

Current	Past History	Other Specified/Unspecified Schizophrenia Spectrum and Other Psychotic Disorder (p. 44/**C30**)
☐	☐	F28 Other Specified: _____
☐	☐	F29 Unspecified

Bipolar and Related Disorders

Current	Past History	Disorder	
		Bipolar I Disorder	
		Bipolar I Disorder, Current or Most Recent Episode Manic (p. 49/**D17**)	
☐		F31.11	Current Episode Manic, Mild
☐		F31.12	Current Episode Manic, Moderate
☐		F31.13	Current Episode Manic, Severe
☐		F31.2	Current Episode Manic, With Psychotic Features
	☐	F31.73	Most Recent Episode Manic, In Partial Remission
	☐	F31.74	Most Recent Episode Manic, In Full Remission
		Bipolar I Disorder, Current or Most Recent Episode Depressed (p. 49/**D18**)	
☐		F31.31	Current Episode Depressed, Mild
☐		F31.32	Current Episode Depressed, Moderate
☐		F31.4	Current Episode Depressed, Severe
☐		F31.5	Current Episode Depressed, With Psychotic Features
	☐	F31.75	Most Recent Episode Depressed, In Partial Remission
	☐	F31.76	Most Recent Episode Depressed, In Full Remission
		Bipolar I Disorder, Current or Most Recent Episode Hypomanic (p. 50/**D19**)	
☐		F31.0	Current Episode Hypomanic
	☐	F31.71	Most Recent Episode Hypomanic, In Partial Remission
	☐	F31.72	Most Recent Episode Hypomanic, In Full Remission
		Bipolar I Disorder, Current or Most Recent Episode Unspecified (p. 50/**D20**)	
☐	☐	F31.9	

---

[1] See page 6 for diagnostic codes for Substance/Medication-Induced Psychotic Disorder.

Current	Past History		Disorder
			Bipolar II Disorder
			Bipolar II Disorder, Current or Most Recent Episode Hypomanic (p. 50/**D21**)
☐		F31.81	Current Episode Hypomanic
	☐	F31.81	Most Recent Episode Hypomanic, In Partial Remission
	☐	F31.81	Most Recent Episode Hypomanic, In Full Remission
			Bipolar II Disorder, Current or Most Recent Episode Depressed (p. 51/**D22**)
☐		F31.81	Current Episode Depressed, Mild
☐		F31.81	Current Episode Depressed, Moderate
☐		F31.81	Current Episode Depressed, Severe
☐		F31.81	Current Episode Depressed, With Psychotic Features
	☐	F31.81	Most Recent Episode Depressed, In Partial Remission
	☐	F31.81	Most Recent Episode Depressed, In Full Remission
	Lifetime		
			Bipolar and Related Disorder Due to Another Medical Condition
			(p. 19/**A40**, p. 22/**A53**, p. 25/**A65**, p. 28/**A77**, p. 47/**D10**)
	☐	F06.33	With Manic Features
	☐	F06.33	With Manic- or Hypomanic-Like Episode
	☐	F06.34	With Mixed Features
			Substance/Medication-Induced Bipolar and Related Disorder
			(p. 19/**A40**, p. 22/**A53**, p. 25/**A65**, p. 28/**A77**, p. 47/**D10**)
	☐	F___.___ [2]	Indicate specific substance and diagnostic code: _____

Current	Past History		
			Other Specified/Unspecified Bipolar and Related Disorder (p. 51/**D23**)
☐	☐	F31.89[3]	Other Specified: _____
☐	☐	F31.9	Unspecified

Depressive Disorders

Current	Past History		Disorder
			Major Depressive Disorder, Single Episode (p. 52/**D24**)
☐		F32.0	Mild (current)
☐		F32.1	Moderate (current)
☐		F32.2	Severe (current)
☐		F32.3	With Psychotic Features (current)
	☐	F32.4	In Partial Remission
	☐	F32.5	In Full Remission
			Major Depressive Disorder, Recurrent Episode (p. 52/**D24**)
☐		F33.0	Mild (current)
☐		F33.1	Moderate (current)
☐		F33.2	Severe (current)
☐		F33.3	With Psychotic Features (current)
	☐	F33.41	In Partial Remission
	☐	F33.42	In Full Remission
			Persistent Depressive Disorder (past 2 years) (p. 30/**A90**)
☐		F34.1	
	Lifetime		
			Depressive Disorder Due to Another Medical Condition (p. 12/**A12**, p. 16/**A26**, p. 30/**A89**, p. 48/**D16**)
	☐	F06.34	With Mixed Features
	☐	F06.31	With Depressive Features
	☐	F06.32	With Major Depressive–Like Episode
			Substance/Medication-Induced Depressive Disorder (p. 12/**A12**, p. 16/**A26**, p. 30/**A89**, p. 48/**D16**)
	☐	F___.___ [4]	Indicate specific substance and diagnostic code: _____

---

[2] See page 6 for diagnostic codes for Substance/Medication-Induced Bipolar Disorder.

[3] The diagnostic code is F34.0 instead of F31.89 if the presentation meets criteria for Cyclothymic Disorder.

[4] See page 6 for diagnostic codes for Substance/Medication-Induced Depressive Disorder.

Current	**Past History**		**Other Specified/Unspecified Depressive Disorder (p. 52/D25)**
☐	☐	F32.89	Other Specified: _____
☐	☐	F32.9	Unspecified

Substance Use Disorders (past 12 months)

Past 12 Months   **Disorder**

Alcohol Use Disorder (p. 55/E13)

☐	F10.10	Mild	
☐	F10.20	Moderate	
☐	F10.20	Severe	

Sedative, Hypnotic, or Anxiolytic Use Disorder (p. 61/E36)   *Specific drug used:* _____

☐	F13.10	Mild	
☐	F13.20	Moderate	
☐	F13.20	Severe	

Cannabis Use Disorder (p. 61/E36)   *Specific drug used:* _____

☐	F12.10	Mild	
☐	F12.20	Moderate	
☐	F12.20	Severe	

Stimulant Use Disorders

Amphetamine-Type Substance Use Disorder (p. 61/E36)   *Specific drug used:* _____

☐	F15.10	Mild	
☐	F15.20	Moderate	
☐	F15.20	Severe	

Cocaine Use Disorder (p. 61/E36)

☐	F14.10	Mild	
☐	F14.20	Moderate	
☐	F14.20	Severe	

Other or Unspecified Stimulant Use Disorder (p. 61/E36)   *Specific drug used:* _____

☐	F15.10	Mild	
☐	F15.20	Moderate	
☐	F15.20	Severe	

Opioid Use Disorder (p. 61/E36)   *Specific drug used:* _____

☐	F11.10	Mild	
☐	F11.20	Moderate	
☐	F11.20	Severe	

Phencyclidine and Related Substance Use Disorder (p. 61/E36)   *Specific drug used:* _____

☐	F16.10	Mild	
☐	F16.20	Moderate	
☐	F16.20	Severe	

Other Hallucinogen Use Disorder (p. 61/E36)   *Specific drug used:* _____

☐	F16.10	Mild	
☐	F16.20	Moderate	
☐	F16.20	Severe	

Inhalant Use Disorder (p. 61/E36)   *Specific drug used:* _____

☐	F18.10	Mild	
☐	F18.20	Moderate	
☐	F18.20	Severe	

Other (or Unknown) Substance Use Disorder (p. 61/E36)   *Specific drug used:* _____

☐	F19.10	Mild	
☐	F19.20	Moderate	
☐	F19.20	Severe	

Other Disorders

Current	Past History	Disorder	
		Panic Disorder (p. 66/ F22)	
☐	☐	F41.0	
		Agoraphobia (past 6 months) (p. 68/F31)	
☐		F40.00	
		Social Anxiety Disorder (past 6 months) (p. 70/F41)	
☐		F40.10	
		Generalized Anxiety Disorder (past 6 months) (p. 72/F54)	
☐		F41.1	
		Obsessive-Compulsive Disorder (past month) (p. 75/G8)	
☐		F42.2	
		Posttraumatic Stress Disorder (p. 85/G41)	
☐	☐	F43.10	
		Attention-Deficit/Hyperactivity Disorder (past 6 months) (p. 90/H26)	
☐		F90.2	Combined Presentation
☐		F90.0	Predominantly Inattentive Presentation
☐		F90.1	Predominantly Hyperactive/Impulsive Presentation
		Adjustment Disorder (past 6 months) (p. 95/J5)	
☐		F43.21	With Depressed Mood
☐		F43.22	With Anxiety
☐		F43.23	With Mixed Anxiety and Depressed Mood
☐		F43.24	With Disturbance of Conduct
☐		F43.25	With Mixed Disturbance of Emotions and Conduct
☐		F43.20	Unspecified

	Lifetime		
		Anxiety Disorder Due to Another Medical Condition (p. 65/F20, p. 70/F39, p. 72/F53)	
	☐	F06.4	
		Substance/Medication-Induced Anxiety Disorder (p. 65/F20, p. 70/F39, p. 72/F53)	
	☐	F___.___ [5] Indicate specific substance and diagnostic code: _____	
		Obsessive-Compulsive and Related Disorder Due to Another Medical Condition (p. 74/G7)	
	☐	F06.8	
		Substance/Medication-Induced Obsessive-Compulsive and Related Disorder (p. 74/G7)	
	☐	F___.___ [6] Indicate specific substance and diagnostic code: _____	

Current	Past History		
☐	☐	F___.___	Other DSM-5 disorder:
☐	☐	F___.___	Other DSM-5 disorder:

---

[5] See page 6 for diagnostic codes for Substance/Medication-Induced Anxiety Disorder.
[6] See page 6 for diagnostic codes for Substance/Medication-Induced Obsessive-Compulsive and Related Disorder.

Screened Disorders (current only)

Current	Disorder
	*Premenstrual Dysphoric Disorder (p. 91/ **I1**)*
☐	*F32.81*
	*Specific Phobia (p. 91/**I2**)*
☐	*F40.218 Animal*
☐	*F40.228 Natural environment*
☐	*F40.230 Fear of blood*
☐	*F40.231 Fear of injections and transfusions*
☐	*F40.232 Fear of other medical care*
☐	*F40.233 Fear of injury*
☐	*F40.248 Situational*
☐	*F40.298 Other*
	*Separation Anxiety Disorder (p. 91/**I3**)*
☐	*F93.0*
	*Hoarding Disorder (p. 91/**I4**)*
☐	*F42.3*
	*Body Dysmorphic Disorder (p. 91/**I5**)*
☐	*F45.22*
	*Trichotillomania (Hair-Pulling Disorder) (p. 91/**I6**)*
☐	*F63.3*
	*Excoriation (Skin-Picking) Disorder (p. 92/**I7**)*
☐	*F42.4*
	*Insomnia Disorder (p. 92/**I8**)*
☐	*F51.01*
	*Hypersomnolence Disorder (p. 92/**I9**)*
☐	*F51.11*
	*Anorexia Nervosa (p. 92/**I10**)*
☐	*F50.01 Restricting type*
☐	*F50.02 Binge-eating/purging type*
	*Bulimia Nervosa (p. 92/**I11**)*
☐	*F50.2*
	*Binge-Eating Disorder (p. 92 (**I11**)*
☐	*F50.81*
	*Avoidant/Restrictive Food Intake Disorder (p. 92/**I12**)*
☐	*F50.82*
	*Somatic Symptom Disorder (p. 92)/**I13**)*
☐	*F45.1*
	*Illness Anxiety Disorder (p. 93/**I14**)*
☐	*F45.21*
	*Intermittent Explosive Disorder (p. 93/**I15**)*
☐	*F63.81*
	*Gambling Disorder (p. 93/**I16**)*
☐	*F63.0*

Diagnostic Codes for Substance/Medication-Induced Psychotic Disorder

Substance class	With use disorder, mild	With use disorder, moderate or severe	Without use disorder
Alcohol	F10.159	F10.259	F10.959
Sedative, hypnotic, or anxiolytic	F13.159	F13.259	F13.959
Cannabis	F12.159	F12.259	F12.959
Amphetamine (or other stimulant)	F15.159	F15.259	F15.959
Cocaine	F14.159	F14.259	F14.959
Phencyclidine	F16.159	F16.259	F16.959
Other hallucinogen	F16.159	F16.259	F16.959
Inhalant	F18.159	F18.259	F18.959
Other (or unknown substance)	F19.159	F19.259	F19.959

Diagnostic Codes for Substance/Medication-Induced Bipolar and Related Disorder

Substance class	With use disorder, mild	With use disorder, moderate or severe	Without use disorder
Alcohol	F10.14	F10.24	F10.94
Sedative, hypnotic, or anxiolytic	F13.14	F13.24	F13.94
Amphetamine (or other stimulant)	F15.14	F15.24	F15.94
Cocaine	F14.14	F14.24	F14.94
Phencyclidine	F16.14	F16.24	F16.94
Other hallucinogen	F16.14	F16.24	F16.94
Other (or unknown substance)	F19.14	F19.24	F19.94

Diagnostic Codes for Substance/Medication-Induced Depressive Disorder

Substance class	With use disorder, mild	With use disorder, moderate or severe	Without use disorder
Alcohol	F10.14	F10.24	F10.94
Sedative, hypnotic, or anxiolytic	F13.14	F13.24	F13.94
Amphetamine (or other stimulant)	F15.14	F15.24	F15.94
Cocaine	F14.14	F14.24	F14.94
Opioid	F11.14	F11.24	F11.94
Phencyclidine	F16.14	F16.24	F16.94
Other hallucinogen	F16.14	F16.24	F16.94
Inhalant	F18.14	F18.24	F18.94
Other (or unknown substance)	F19.14	F19.24	F19.94

Diagnostic Codes for Substance/Medication-Induced Anxiety Disorder

Substance class	With use disorder, mild	With use disorder, moderate or severe	Without use disorder
Alcohol	F10.180	F10.280	F10.980
Sedative, hypnotic, or anxiolytic	F13.180	F13.280	F13.980
Cannabis	F12.180	F12.280	F12.980
Amphetamine (or other stimulant)	F15.180	F15.280	F15.980
Cocaine	F14.180	F14.280	F14.980
Caffeine	—	—	F15.980
Opioid	F11.188	F11.288	F11.988
Phencyclidine	F16.180	F16.280	F16.980
Other hallucinogen	F16.180	F16.280	F16.980
Inhalant	F18.180	F18.280	F18.980
Other (or unknown substance)	F19.180	F19.280	F19.980

Diagnostic Codes for Substance/Medication-Induced Obsessive-Compulsive and Related Disorder

Substance class	With use disorder, mild	With use disorder, moderate or severe	Without use disorder
Amphetamine (or other stimulant)	F15.188	F15.288	F15.988
Cocaine	F14.188	F14.288	F14.988
Other (or unknown substance)	F19.188	F19.288	F19.988

OVERVIEW

I'm going to be asking you about problems or difficulties you may have had, and I'll be making some notes as we go along. Do you have any questions before we begin?

How old are you?

With whom do you live? (What kind of place do you live in?)

What kind of work do you do?

Have you always done that kind of work?

Are you currently employed (getting paid)?

> IF YES: **Do you work part-time or full-time?**

>> IF PART-TIME: **How many hours do you typically work each week? (Why do you work part-time instead of full-time?)**

> IF NO: **Why is that? When was the last time you worked? How are you supporting yourself now?**

>> IF DISABLED: **Are you currently receiving disability payments? Why are you on disability?**

IF UNKNOWN: **Has there ever been a period of time when you were unable to work or go to school?**

> IF YES: **Why was that?**

HISTORY OF CURRENT ILLNESS

What led to your coming here (this time)? (What's the major problem you've been having trouble with?)

What was going on in your life when this began?

When were you last feeling OK (your usual self)?

TREATMENT HISTORY

NOTE: The goal of this section of the Overview is to determine the overall "landscape" of the person's lifetime psychopathology. Avoid going into excessive detail. For major past episodes, determine symptoms, medications, other treatments ("What treatment did you get for that?"), and approximate onset and offset ("When did it start? When were you feeling better?").

When was the first time you saw someone for emotional or psychiatric problems? (What was that for? What treatment[s] did you get? What medications?)

Have you ever been a patient in a psychiatric hospital?

> IF YES: **What was that for? (How many times?)**

> IF AN INADEQUATE ANSWER IS GIVEN, CHALLENGE GENTLY—e.g., **Wasn't there something else? People don't usually go to psychiatric hospitals just because they are (tired/nervous/OWN WORDS).**

Have you ever had any treatment for drugs or alcohol?

Age (or date)	Description (symptoms, triggering events)	Treatment and offset
_____	_____	_____
_____	_____	_____
_____	_____	_____

Continue treatment history on page 9 if necessary.

MEDICAL PROBLEMS

How has your physical health been? (Have you had any medical problems?)

Have you ever been in a hospital for treatment of a medical problem? (What was that for?)

Do you take any medications, vitamins, or other nutritional supplements (other than those you've already told me about)?

    IF YES: **What are you taking and at what dose?**

SUICIDAL IDEATION AND BEHAVIOR

CHECK FOR THOUGHTS: **Have you ever wished you were dead or wished you could go to sleep and not wake up? (Tell me about that.)**

➤IF NO: SKIP TO **SUICIDE ATTEMPT,** BELOW.

➤IF YES: **Did you have any of these thoughts in the past week (including today)?**

    ➤IF NO: SKIP TO **SUICIDE ATTEMPT,** BELOW.

    ➤IF YES: CHECK FOR INTENT: **Have you had a strong urge to kill yourself at any time in the past week? (Tell me about that.)
In the past week, did you have any intention of attempting suicide? (Tell me about that.)**

CHECK FOR PLAN AND METHOD: **In the past week, have you thought about <u>how</u> you might actually do it? (Tell me about what you were thinking of doing.) Have you thought about what you would need to do to carry this out? (Tell me about that. Do you have the means to do this?)**

SUICIDE ATTEMPT

CHECK FOR ATTEMPT: **Have you ever tried to kill yourself?**

➤ IF NO: **Have you ever done anything to harm yourself?**

    IF NO, GO TO **OTHER CURRENT PROBLEMS,** BELOW.

➤ IF YES: **What did you do? (Tell me what happened.) Were you trying to end your life?**

IF MORE THAN ONE ATTEMPT: **Which attempt had the most severe medical consequences (going to the emergency department, needing hospitalization, requiring care in ICU)?**

Have you made any suicide attempts in the past week (including today)?

OTHER CURRENT PROBLEMS

Have you had any other problems in the past month? (How are things going at work, at home, and with other people?)

What has your mood been like?

In the past month, how much have you been drinking?

When you drink, who are you usually with? (Are you usually alone or out with other people?)

In the past month, have you been using any illegal or recreational drugs? How about taking more of your prescription drugs than was prescribed or running out of medication early?

TREATMENT HISTORY *(continued)*

Age (or date)	Description (symptoms, triggering events)	Treatment and offset
_____	_____	_____
_____	_____	_____
_____	_____	_____
_____	_____	_____
_____	_____	_____
_____	_____	_____
_____	_____	_____
_____	_____	_____
_____	_____	_____
_____	_____	_____
_____	_____	_____
_____	_____	_____
_____	_____	_____
_____	_____	_____
_____	_____	_____
_____	_____	_____
_____	_____	_____
_____	_____	_____
_____	_____	_____

A. MOOD EPISODES

	CURRENT MAJOR DEPRESSIVE EPISODE	MAJOR DEPRESSIVE EPISODE CRITERIA			
	Now I am going to ask you some more questions about your mood.	A. Five (or more) of the following symptoms have been present during the same 2-week period and represent a change from previous functioning; at least one of the symptoms is either (1) depressed mood or (2) loss of interest or pleasure.			
A1	In the past month, since (ONE MONTH AGO), has there been a period of time when you were feeling depressed or down most of the day, <u>nearly every day</u>? (Has anyone said that you look sad, down, or depressed?) IF NO: <u>How about feeling sad, empty, or hopeless, most of the day, nearly every day?</u> IF YES TO EITHER OF ABOVE: **What has it been like? How long has it lasted? (As long as 2 weeks?)**	1. Depressed mood most of the day, nearly every day, as indicated by either subjective report (e.g., feels sad, empty, hopeless) or observation made by others (e.g., appears tearful).	—	+	A1
A2	▶ IF PREVIOUS ITEM RATED "+": **During that time, did you have less interest or pleasure in things you usually enjoyed? (What has that been like?)** ▶ IF PREVIOUS ITEM RATED "—": **What about a time since (ONE MONTH AGO) when you lost interest or pleasure in things you usually enjoyed? (What has that been like?)** IF YES TO EITHER OF ABOVE: <u>Has it been nearly every day?</u> **How long has it lasted? (As long as 2 weeks?)**	2. Markedly diminished interest or pleasure in all, or almost all, activities most of the day, nearly every day (as indicated by either subjective account or observation).	—	+	A2

> **IF BOTH A1 AND A2 ARE RATED AS "—" FOR THE CURRENT MONTH, Continue with A15 (Past Major Depressive Episode), page 13.**

	FOR THE FOLLOWING QUESTIONS, FOCUS ON THE WORST 2-WEEK PERIOD OF THE PAST MONTH: **During (2-WEEK PERIOD)...**				
A3	**...how has your appetite been? (What about compared to your usual appetite? Have you had to force yourself to eat? Eat [less/more] than usual? <u>Has that been nearly every day?</u> Have you lost or gained any weight?)** IF YES: **How much? (Had you been trying to [lose/gain] weight?)**	3. Significant weight loss when not dieting or weight gain (e.g., a change of more than 5% of body weight in a month), or decrease or increase in appetite nearly every day.	—	+	A3

A4	...how have you bee*n* sleeping? (Trouble falling asleep, waking frequently, trouble staying asleep, waking too early, OR sleeping too much?) How many hours of sleep (including naps) have you been getting? How many hours of sleep did you typically get before you got (depressed/OWN WORDS)? <u>Has it been nearly every night?</u>	4. Insomnia or hypersomnia nearly every day.	—	+	A4
A5	...have you been so fidgety or restless that you were unable to sit still? What about the opposite—talking more slowly, or moving more slowly than is normal for you, as if you're moving through molasses or mud? (In either instance, has it been so bad that other people have noticed it? What have they noticed? <u>Has that been nearly every day?</u>)	5. Psychomotor agitation or retardation nearly every day (observable by others, not merely subjective feelings of restlessness or being slowed down). *NOTE: CONSIDER BEHAVIOR DURING THE INTERVIEW.*	—	+	A5
A6	...what was your energy like? (Tired all the time? <u>Nearly every day?</u>)	6. Fatigue or loss of energy nearly every day.	—	+	A6
A7	...have you been feeling worthless? What about feeling guilty about things you have done or not done? IF YES: What kinds of things? (Is this only because you can't take care of things since you have been sick?) IF YES TO EITHER OF ABOVE: <u>Nearly every day?</u>	7. Feelings of worthlessness or excessive or inappropriate guilt (which may be delusional) nearly every day (not merely self-reproach or guilt about being sick).	—	+	A7
A8	...have you had trouble thinking or concentrating? Has it been hard to make decisions about everyday things? (What kinds of things has it been interfering with? <u>Nearly every day?</u>)	8. Diminished ability to think or concentrate, or indecisiveness, nearly every day (either by subjective account or as observed by others).	—	+	A8
A9	...have things been so bad that you thought a lot about death or that you would be better off dead? Have you thought about taking your own life? IF YES: Have you done something about it? (What have you done? Have you made a specific plan? Have you taken any action to prepare for it? Have you actually made a suicide attempt?)	9. Recurrent thoughts of death (not just fear of dying), recurrent suicidal ideation without a specific plan, or a suicide attempt or a specific plan for committing suicide.	—	+	A9
A10		AT LEAST FIVE OF THE ABOVE CRITERION A SXS **(A1–A9)** ARE RATED "+".	**NO** ↓ Continue with **A15** (Past Major Depressive Episode), **page 13.**	**YES** ↓ Continue with **A11, next page.**	A1

| **A11** | IF UNCLEAR: **What effect have** (DEPRESSIVE SXS) **had on your life?** | B. The symptoms cause clinically significant distress or impairment in social, occupational, or other important areas of functioning. | −   + | **A11** |

ASK THE FOLLOWING QUESTIONS ONLY AS NEEDED:

How have (DEPRESSIVE SXS) **affected your relationships or your interactions with other people? (Have** [DEPRESSIVE SXS] **caused you any problems in your relationships with your family, romantic partner, or friends?)**

How have (DEPRESSIVE SXS) **affected your work/school? (How about your attendance at work/school? Have** [DEPRESSIVE SXS] **made it more difficult to do your work/schoolwork? Have** [DEPRESSIVE SXS] **affected the quality of your work/schoolwork?)**

How have (DEPRESSIVE SXS) **affected your ability to take care of things at home? How about doing simple everyday things, like getting dressed, bathing, or brushing your teeth? What about doing other things that are important to you, like religious activities, physical exercise, or hobbies? Have you avoided doing anything because you felt like you weren't up to it?**

Have (DEPRESSIVE SXS) **affected any other important part of your life?**

IF DEPRESSIVE SXS DO NOT INTERFERE WITH LIFE: **How much have you been bothered or upset by having** (DEPRESSIVE SXS)**?**

Continue with **A12**, below.

Continue with **A15** (Past Major Depressive Episode), **page 13.**

| **A12** | IF UNKNOWN: **When did** (EPISODE OF DEPRESSION) **begin?** | C. [Primary Depressive Episode] The episode is not attributable to the physiological effects of a substance [e.g., a drug of abuse, medication] or another medical condition. | **NO**   **YES** | **A12** |

Just before this period of depression began, were you physically ill?

   IF YES: **What did the doctor say?**

Just before this began, were you taking any medications?

   IF YES: **Any change in the amount you were taking?**

Just before this began, were you drinking or using any street drugs?

> Refer to the User's Guide, Section 9, for guidance on determining whether there is an etiological GMC or substance/medication.

NOTE: *Code "NO" only if episode is due to a GMC or substance/medication.*

Etiological GMCs include stroke, Huntington's disease, Parkinson's disease, traumatic brain injury, Cushing's disease, hypothyroidism, multiple sclerosis, systemic lupus erythematosus.

Etiological substances/medications include alcohol (I/W); phencyclidine (I); hallucinogens (I); inhalants (I); opioids (I/W); sedatives, hypnotics, or anxiolytics (I/W); amphetamine and other stimulants (I/W); cocaine (I/W); antiviral agents (efavirenz); cardiovascular agents (clonidine, guanethidine, methyldopa, reserpine); retinoic acid derivatives (isotretinoin); antidepressants; anticonvulsants; anti-migraine agents (triptans); antipsychotics; hormonal agents (corticosteroids, oral contraceptives, gonadotropin-releasing hormone agonists, tamoxifen); smoking cessation agents (varenicline); and immunological agents (interferon).

PRIMARY

Diagnose: Depressive Disorder Due to AMC or Substance-Induced Depressive Disorder

Continue with **A15** (Past Major Depressive Episode), **page 13.**

CURRENT MAJOR DEPRESSIVE EPISODE Continue with **A13**, next page.

A13	IF UNKNOWN: **When did this period of (depression/OWN WORDS) begin?**	Onset of depression (month/year)
		___ / ___ A1

A14	**How many separate times in your life have you been (depressed/ OWN WORDS) nearly every day for at least 2 weeks and had several of the symptoms that you described, like (SXS OF CURRENT MAJOR DEPRESSIVE EPISODE)?**	Total number of Major Depressive Episodes, including current (CODE 99 IF TOO NUMEROUS OR INDISTINCT TO COUNT).
		___ ___ A1
		↓ Continue with **A29** (Current Manic Episode), **page 17.**

	PAST MAJOR DEPRESSIVE EPISODE	MAJOR DEPRESSIVE EPISODE CRITERIA		
	NOTE: IF THERE IS CURRENTLY DEPRESSED MOOD OR LOSS OF INTEREST BUT FULL CRITERIA ARE NOT MET FOR A MAJOR DEPRESSIVE EPISODE, SUBSTITUTE THE PHRASE **"Has there ever been another time..."** *IN EACH OF THE TWO SCREENING QUESTIONS BELOW (I.E., A15 AND A16).*	A. Five (or more) of the following symptoms have been present during the same 2-week period and represent a change from previous functioning; at least one of the symptoms is either (1) depressed mood, or (2) loss of interest or pleasure.		
A15	**Have you <u>ever</u> had a period of time when you were feeling depressed or down most of the day, <u>nearly every day</u>? (What was that like?)** IF NO: **How about feeling sad, empty, or hopeless, most of the day, nearly every day?** IF YES TO EITHER OF ABOVE: **How long did it last? (As long as 2 weeks?)**	1. Depressed mood most of the day, nearly every day, as indicated by either subjective report (e.g., feels sad, empty, hopeless) or observation made by others (e.g., appears tearful).	− +	A
A16	▶ IF PREVIOUS ITEM RATED "+": **During that time, did you lose interest or pleasure in things you usually enjoyed? (What was that like?)** ↳ IF PREVIOUS ITEM RATED "—": **Have you <u>ever</u> had a period of time when you lost interest or pleasure in things you usually enjoyed? (What was that like?)** IF YES TO EITHER OF ABOVE: **When was that? <u>Was it nearly every day?</u> How long did it last? (As long as 2 weeks?)**	2. Markedly diminished interest or pleasure in all, or almost all, activities most of the day, nearly every day (as indicated by either subjective account or observation).	− +	A

IF BOTH A15 AND A16 ARE RATED AS "—", continue with A29 (Current Manic Episode), page 17.

Have you had more than one time like that? (Which time was the worst?) IF UNCLEAR: **Have you had any times like that since (ONE YEAR AGO)?**	*NOTE: If more than one past episode is likely, select the "worst" one for your inquiry about a past Major Depressive Episode. However, if there was an episode in the past year, ask about that episode even if it was not the worst.*

FOR THE FOLLOWING QUESTIONS, FOCUS ON THE WORST 2 WEEKS OF THE PAST MAJOR DEPRESSIVE EPISODE THAT YOU ARE INQUIRING ABOUT.

     IF UNCLEAR: **During** (MAJOR DEPRESSIVE EPISODE) **when were you the most (depressed/OWN WORDS)?**

A17	**During** (WORST 2-WEEK PERIOD)… …**how was your appetite? (What about compared to your usual appetite? Did you have to force yourself to eat? Eat [less/more] than usual? <u>Was that nearly every day?</u> Did you lose or gain any weight? (How much? Were you trying to lose or gain weight?)**	3. Significant weight loss when not dieting or weight gain (e.g., a change of more than 5% of body weight in a month), or decrease or increase in appetite nearly every day.	—	+	**A17**
A18	…**how were you sleeping? (Trouble falling asleep, waking frequently, trouble staying asleep, waking too early, OR sleeping too much?)** **How many hours of sleep (including naps) had you been getting? How many hours of sleep did you typically get before you got (depressed/OWN WORDS)? <u>Was that nearly every night?</u>**	4. Insomnia or hypersomnia nearly every day.	—	+	**A18**
A19	…**Were you so fidgety or restless that you were unable to sit still?** **What about the opposite—talking more slowly, or moving more slowly than is normal for you, as if you were moving through molasses or mud?** **(In either instance, was it so bad that other people noticed it? What did they notice? <u>Was that nearly every day?</u>)**	5. Psychomotor agitation or retardation nearly every day (observable by others, not merely subjective feelings of restlessness or being slowed down). *NOTE: CONSIDER BEHAVIOR DURING THE INTERVIEW.*	—	+	**A19**
A20	…**what was your energy like? (Tired all the time? <u>Nearly every day?</u>)**	6. Fatigue or loss of energy nearly every day.	—	+	**A20**
A21	…**Were you feeling worthless?** **What about feeling guilty about things you had done or not done?** IF YES: **What kinds of things? (Was this only because you couldn't take care of things since you had been sick?)** IF YES TO EITHER OF ABOVE: <u>**Nearly every day?**</u>	7. Feelings of worthlessness or excessive or inappropriate guilt (which may be delusional) nearly every day (not merely self-reproach or guilt about being sick).	—	+	**A21**
A22	…**did you have trouble thinking or concentrating? Was it hard to make decisions about everyday things? (What kinds of things was it interfering with? <u>Nearly every day?</u>)**	8. Diminished ability to think or concentrate, or indecisiveness, nearly every day (either by subjective account or as observed by others).	—	+	**A22**

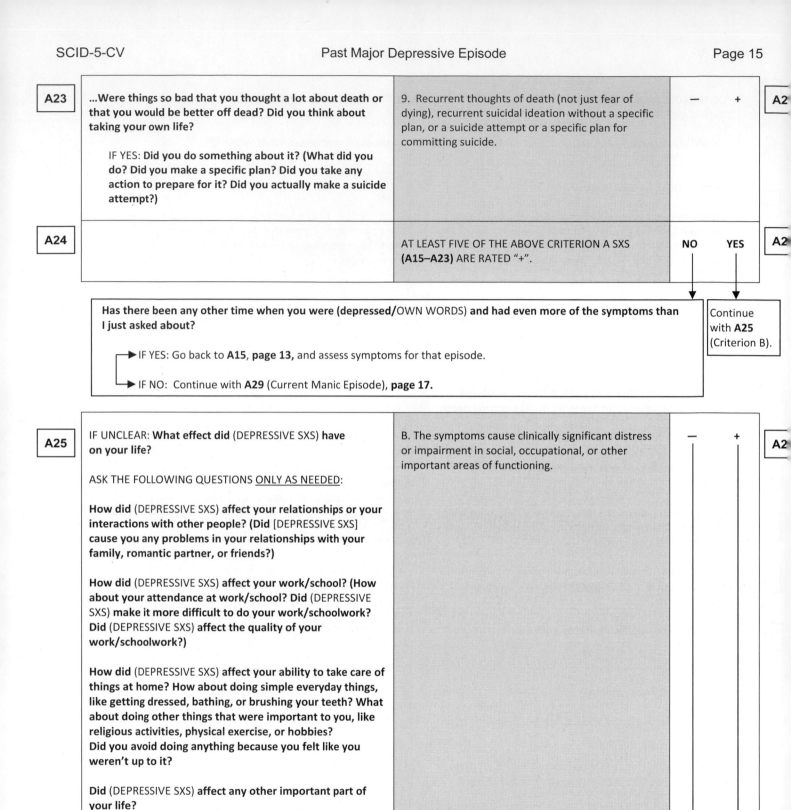

A23

...Were things so bad that you thought a lot about death or that you would be better off dead? Did you think about taking your own life?

IF YES: **Did you do something about it? (What did you do? Did you make a specific plan? Did you take any action to prepare for it? Did you actually make a suicide attempt?)**

9. Recurrent thoughts of death (not just fear of dying), recurrent suicidal ideation without a specific plan, or a suicide attempt or a specific plan for committing suicide.

—   +

A2

A24

AT LEAST FIVE OF THE ABOVE CRITERION A SXS **(A15–A23)** ARE RATED "+".

NO   YES

A2

Has there been any other time when you were (depressed/OWN WORDS**) and had even more of the symptoms than I just asked about?**

➤ IF YES: Go back to **A15**, **page 13,** and assess symptoms for that episode.

➤ IF NO: Continue with **A29** (Current Manic Episode), **page 17.**

Continue with **A25** (Criterion B).

A25

IF UNCLEAR: **What effect did** (DEPRESSIVE SXS) **have on your life?**

ASK THE FOLLOWING QUESTIONS <u>ONLY AS NEEDED</u>:

How did (DEPRESSIVE SXS) **affect your relationships or your interactions with other people? (Did** [DEPRESSIVE SXS] **cause you any problems in your relationships with your family, romantic partner, or friends?)**

How did (DEPRESSIVE SXS) **affect your work/school? (How about your attendance at work/school? Did** (DEPRESSIVE SXS) **make it more difficult to do your work/schoolwork? Did** (DEPRESSIVE SXS) **affect the quality of your work/schoolwork?)**

How did (DEPRESSIVE SXS) **affect your ability to take care of things at home? How about doing simple everyday things, like getting dressed, bathing, or brushing your teeth? What about doing other things that were important to you, like religious activities, physical exercise, or hobbies? Did you avoid doing anything because you felt like you weren't up to it?**

Did (DEPRESSIVE SXS) **affect any other important part of your life?**

IF DEPRESSIVE SXS DID NOT INTERFERE WITH LIFE: **How much were you bothered or upset by having** (DEPRESSIVE SXS)**?**

B. The symptoms cause clinically significant distress or impairment in social, occupational, or other important areas of functioning.

—   +

A2

Has there been any other time when you were (depressed/OWN WORDS**) and it caused even more problems than the time I just asked about?**

➤ IF YES: Go back to **A15**, **page 13,** and assess symptoms for that episode.

➤ IF NO: Continue with **A29** (Current Manic Episode), **page 17.**

Continue with **A26** (Criterion C), **next page.**

A26	IF UNKNOWN: **When did** (EPISODE OF DEPRESSION) **begin?**
	
	Just before this began, were you physically ill?
	
	   IF YES: **What did the doctor say?**
	
	Just before this began, were you taking any medications?
	
	   IF YES: **Any change in the amount you were taking?**
	
	Just before this began, were you drinking or using any street drugs?
	
	Refer to the User's Guide, Section 9, for guidance on determining whether there is an etiological GMC or substance/medication.
		C. [Primary Depressive Episode] The episode is not attributable to the physiological effects of a substance (e.g., a drug of abuse, medication) or another medical condition.
		
		NOTE: Code "NO" only if episode is due to a GMC or substance/medication.
		
		Refer to list of etiological GMCs and substances/medications in A12, page 12.
			NO YES → PRIMARY
			
			↓ Diagnose: Depressive Disorder Due to AMC or Substance-Induced Depressive Disorder
			
			→ **PAST MAJOR DEPRESSIVE EPISODE**
				A26

IF UNKNOWN: **Has there been any other time when you were (depressed/OWN WORDS) like this but were not (ill with GMC/using SUBSTANCE)?**

    → IF YES: Go back to **A15**, **page 13**, and assess symptoms for that episode.

    → IF NO: Continue with **A29** (Current Manic Episode), **page 17**.

Continue with **A27**, below.

A27	IF UNKNOWN: **When did this period of (depression/OWN WORDS) begin?**	Onset of depression (month/year)	___/___	A27
A28	**How many separate times in your life have you been (depressed/ OWN WORDS) nearly every day for at least 2 weeks and had several of the symptoms that you described, like (SXS OF WORST EPISODE)?**	Total number of Major Depressive Episodes, including current (CODE 99 IF TOO NUMEROUS OR INDISTINCT TO COUNT.)	__ __ Continue with **A29** (Current Manic Episode), **next page.**	A28

	CURRENT MANIC EPISODE	MANIC EPISODE CRITERIA	
A29	In the past month, since (ONE MONTH AGO), has there been a period of time when you were feeling so good, "high," excited, or "on top of the world" that other people thought you were not your normal self? ▶ IF YES: **What has it been like? (More than just feeling good?)** Have you also been feeling like you were "hyper" or "wired" and had an unusual amount of energy? Have you been much more active than is typical for you? (Have other people commented on how much you have been doing?)		
	▶ IF NO: **Since** (ONE MONTH AGO), **have you had a period of time when you were feeling irritable, angry, or short-tempered for most of the day, for at least several days?** (Is that different from the way you usually are?) **What has it been like?** Have you also been feeling like you were "hyper" or "wired" and had an unusual amount of energy? Have you been much more active than is typical for you? (Have other people commented on how much you were doing?)	A. A distinct period [lasting at least several days] of abnormally and persistently elevated, expansive, or irritable mood and abnormally and persistently increased activity or energy.	— + **A2** Continue with **A54** (Past Manic Episode), **page 22.**
A30	How long has this lasted? (As long as 1 week?) IF LESS THAN 1 WEEK: **Did you need to go into the hospital to protect you from hurting yourself or someone else, or from doing something that could have caused serious financial or legal problems?** Have you been feeing (high/irritable/OWN WORDS) for most of the day, <u>nearly every day,</u> during this time?	...lasting at least 1 week and present most of the day, nearly every day (or any duration if hospitalization is necessary). *NOTE: IF ELEVATED MOOD LASTS LESS THAN 1 WEEK, CHECK WHETHER THERE HAS BEEN A PERIOD OF IRRITABLE MOOD LASTING AT LEAST 1 WEEK BEFORE SKIPPING TO A41.*	— + **A3** Continue with **A41** (Current Hypomanic Episode), **page 20.**
	FOR **A31–A37**, FOCUS ON THE MOST SEVERE WEEK IN THE PAST MONTH OF THE CURRENT EPISODE. IF UNKNOWN: **During** (EPISODE), **when were you the most** (high/irritable/OWN WORDS)?	B. During the period of mood disturbance and increased energy or activity, three (or more) of the following symptoms (four if the mood is only irritable) are present to a significant degree and represent a noticeable change from usual behavior:	
A31	During that time... ...how did you feel about yourself? (More self-confident than usual? Did you feel much smarter or better than everyone else? Did you feel like you had any special powers or abilities?)	1. Inflated self-esteem or grandiosity.	— + **A3**

A32	...did you need less sleep than usual? (How much sleep did you get?) IF YES: **Did you still feel rested?**	2. Decreased need for sleep (e.g., feels rested after only 3 hours of sleep).	−	+	**A32**
A33	...were you much more talkative than usual? (Did people have trouble stopping you or understanding you? Did people have trouble getting a word in edgewise?)	3. More talkative than usual or pressure to keep talking.	−	+	**A33**
A34	...were your thoughts racing through your head? (What was that like?)	4. Flight of ideas or subjective experience that thoughts are racing.	−	+	**A34**
A35	...were you so easily distracted by things around you that you had trouble concentrating or staying on one track? (Give me an example of that.)	5. Distractibility (i.e., attention too easily drawn to unimportant or irrelevant external stimuli), as reported or observed.	−	+	**A35**
A36	...how did you spend your time? (Work, friends, hobbies? Were you especially busy during that time?) (Did you find yourself more enthusiastic at work or working harder at your job? Did you find yourself more engaged in school activities or studying harder?) (Were you more sociable during that time, such as calling on friends, going out with them more than you usually do, or making a lot of new friends?) (Were you spending more time thinking about sex or involved in doing something sexual, by yourself or with others? Was that a big change for you?) Were you physically restless during this time, doing things like pacing a lot, or being unable to sit still? (How bad was it?)	6. Increase in goal-directed activity (either socially, at work or school, or sexually) or psychomotor agitation (i.e., purposeless non-goal-directed activity).	−	+	**A36**
A37	...were you doing anything that could have caused trouble for you or your family? (Spending money on things you didn't need or couldn't afford? How about giving away money or valuable things? Gambling with money you couldn't afford to lose?) (Anything sexual that was likely to get you in trouble? Driving recklessly?) (Did you make any risky or impulsive business investments or get involved in a business scheme that you wouldn't normally have done?)	7. Excessive involvement in activities that have a high potential for painful consequences (e.g., engaging in unrestrained buying sprees, sexual indiscretions, or foolish business investments).	−	+	**A37**

A38		AT LEAST THREE OF THE ABOVE CRITERION B SXS **(A31–A37)** ARE RATED "+" (FOUR IF MOOD ONLY IRRITABLE).	**NO** → Continue with **A54** (Past Manic Episode), **page 22.** **YES** → Continue with **A39**, CRITERION C. **A3**

A39	IF UNCLEAR: **What effect have (MANIC SXS) had on your life?** IF UNKNOWN: **Have you needed to go into the hospital to protect you from hurting yourself or someone else, or from doing something that could have caused serious financial or legal problems?** ASK THE FOLLOWING QUESTIONS <u>ONLY AS NEEDED</u>: **How have (MANIC SXS) affected your relationships or your interactions with other people? (Have [MANIC SXS] caused you any problems in your relationships with your family, romantic partner, or friends?)** **How have (MANIC SXS) affected your work/school? (How about your attendance at work/school? Have [MANIC SXS] made it more difficult to do your work/schoolwork? Have [MANIC SXS] affected the quality of your work/schoolwork?)** **How have (MANIC SXS) affected your ability to take care of things at home?**	C. The mood disturbance is sufficiently severe to cause marked impairment in social or occupational functioning or to necessitate hospitalization to prevent harm to self or others, or there are psychotic features.	**–** **+** **A3** ↓ Continue with **A50** (Current Hypomanic Episode, Criterion C), **page 21.**

A40	IF UNKNOWN: **When did this period of being (high/irritable/OWN WORDS) begin?**
	
	Just before this began, were you physically ill?
	
	  IF YES: **What did the doctor say?**
	
	Just before this began, were you taking any medications?
	
	  IF YES: **Any change in the amount you were taking?**
	
	Just before this began, were you drinking or using any street drugs?
	
	  ⌐ Refer to the User's Guide, Section 9, for guidance on determining whether there is an etiological GMC or substance/medication. ⌐
		D. [Primary Manic Episode] The episode is not attributable to the physiological effects of a substance (e.g., a drug of abuse, a medication, other treatment) or another medical condition.
		
		Note: A full Manic Episode that emerges during antidepressant treatment (e.g., medication, electroconvulsive therapy) but persists at a fully syndromal level beyond the physiological effect of that treatment is sufficient evidence for a Manic Episode and, therefore, a Bipolar I [Disorder] diagnosis.
		
		NOTE: Code "NO" only if episode is due to a GMC or substance/medication.
		
		<u>Etiological GMCs include</u> Alzheimer's disease, vascular dementia, HIV-induced dementia, Huntington's disease, Lewy body disease, Wernicke-Korsakoff syndrome, Cushing's disease, multiple sclerosis, amyotrophic lateral sclerosis, Parkinson's disease, Pick's disease, Creutzfeldt-Jakob disease, stroke, traumatic brain injuries, and hyperthyroidism.
		
		<u>Etiological substances/medications include</u> alcohol (I/W); phencyclidine (I); hallucinogens (I); sedatives, hypnotics, and anxiolytics (I/W); amphetamines (I/W); cocaine (I/W); corticosteroids; androgens; isoniazid; levodopa; interferon-alpha; varenicline; procarbazine; clarithromycin; and ciprofloxacin.
			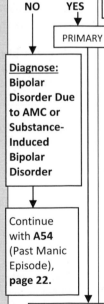 **NO** **YES** **A4**
			↓ PRIMARY
			Diagnose: **Bipolar Disorder Due to AMC or Substance-Induced Bipolar Disorder**
			↓
			Continue with **A54** (Past Manic Episode), **page 22.**
			
			CURRENT MANIC EPISODE Continue with **B1** (Psychotic Symptoms), **page 31.**

	CURRENT HYPOMANIC EPISODE	HYPOMANIC EPISODE CRITERIA		
A41	Has the period when you were feeling (high/irritable/OWN WORDS) lasted for at least 4 days? <u>Has it lasted for most of the day, nearly every day?</u> Have you had more than one time like that since (ONE MONTH AGO)? (Which one was the most extreme?)	A. A distinct period of abnormally and persistently elevated, expansive, or irritable mood and abnormally and persistently increased activity or energy, lasting at least 4 consecutive days and present most of the day, nearly every day.	− + ↓ Continue with **A54** (Past Manic Episode), **page 22.**	A41
	FOR **A42–A48**, FOCUS ON THE MOST EXTREME PERIOD IN THE PAST MONTH OF THE CURRENT EPISODE. IF UNKNOWN: **During (EPISODE), when were you the most (high/irritable/OWN WORDS)?**	B. During the period of mood disturbance and increased energy and activity, three (or more) of the following symptoms (four if the mood is only irritable) have persisted, represent a noticeable change from usual behavior, and have been present to a significant degree:		
A42	During that time… …how were you feeling about yourself? (More self-confident than usual? Did you feel much smarter or better than everyone else? Did you feel like you had any special powers or abilities?)	1. Inflated self-esteem or grandiosity.	− +	A42
A43	…did you need less sleep than usual? (How much sleep did you get?) IF YES: Were you still feeling rested?	2. Decreased need for sleep (e.g., feels rested after only 3 hours of sleep).	− +	A43
A44	…were you much more talkative than usual? (Did people have trouble stopping you, understanding you, or getting a word in edgewise?)	3. More talkative than usual or pressure to keep talking.	− +	A44
A45	…were your thoughts racing through your head? (What was that like?)	4. Flight of ideas or subjective experience that thoughts are racing.	− +	A45
A46	…were you so easily distracted by things around you that you had trouble concentrating or staying on one track? (Give me an example of that.)	5. Distractibility (i.e., attention too easily drawn to unimportant or irrelevant external stimuli), as reported or observed.	− +	A46
A47	…how were you spending your time? (Work, friends, hobbies? Were you especially productive or busy during that time?) (Were you finding yourself more enthusiastic at work or working harder at your job? Did you find yourself more engaged in school activities or studying harder?) (Were you more sociable during that time, such as calling on friends, going out with them more than you usually do, or making a lot of new friends?) (Were you spending more time thinking about sex or involved in doing something sexual, by yourself or with others? Was that a big change for you?) Were you physically restless during this time, doing things like pacing a lot or being unable to sit still? (How bad was it?)	6. Increase in goal-directed activity (either socially, at work or school, or sexually) or psychomotor agitation.	− +	A47

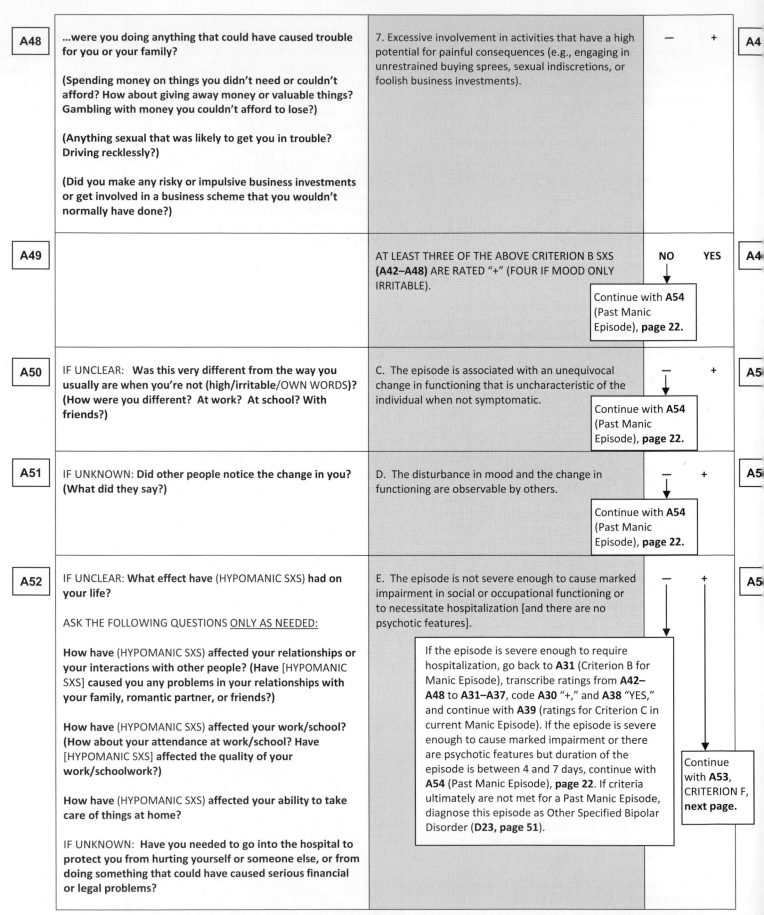

A48	...were you doing anything that could have caused trouble for you or your family? (Spending money on things you didn't need or couldn't afford? How about giving away money or valuable things? Gambling with money you couldn't afford to lose?) (Anything sexual that was likely to get you in trouble? Driving recklessly?) (Did you make any risky or impulsive business investments or get involved in a business scheme that you wouldn't normally have done?)	7. Excessive involvement in activities that have a high potential for painful consequences (e.g., engaging in unrestrained buying sprees, sexual indiscretions, or foolish business investments).	— +	A4
A49		AT LEAST THREE OF THE ABOVE CRITERION B SXS **(A42–A48)** ARE RATED "+" (FOUR IF MOOD ONLY IRRITABLE).	NO YES ↓ Continue with **A54** (Past Manic Episode), **page 22.**	A4
A50	IF UNCLEAR: Was this very different from the way you usually are when you're not (high/irritable/OWN WORDS)? (How were you different? At work? At school? With friends?)	C. The episode is associated with an unequivocal change in functioning that is uncharacteristic of the individual when not symptomatic.	— + ↓ Continue with **A54** (Past Manic Episode), **page 22.**	A5
A51	IF UNKNOWN: **Did other people notice the change in you?** (What did they say?)	D. The disturbance in mood and the change in functioning are observable by others.	— + ↓ Continue with **A54** (Past Manic Episode), **page 22.**	A5
A52	IF UNCLEAR: **What effect have** (HYPOMANIC SXS) **had on your life?** ASK THE FOLLOWING QUESTIONS <u>ONLY AS NEEDED:</u> **How have** (HYPOMANIC SXS) **affected your relationships or your interactions with other people?** (Have [HYPOMANIC SXS] caused you any problems in your relationships with your family, romantic partner, or friends?) **How have** (HYPOMANIC SXS) **affected your work/school?** (How about your attendance at work/school? Have [HYPOMANIC SXS] **affected the quality of your work/schoolwork?**) **How have** (HYPOMANIC SXS) **affected your ability to take care of things at home?** IF UNKNOWN: **Have you needed to go into the hospital to protect you from hurting yourself or someone else, or from doing something that could have caused serious financial or legal problems?**	E. The episode is not severe enough to cause marked impairment in social or occupational functioning or to necessitate hospitalization [and there are no psychotic features]. If the episode is severe enough to require hospitalization, go back to **A31** (Criterion B for Manic Episode), transcribe ratings from **A42–A48** to **A31–A37**, code **A30** "+," and **A38** "YES," and continue with **A39** (ratings for Criterion C in current Manic Episode). If the episode is severe enough to cause marked impairment or there are psychotic features but duration of the episode is between 4 and 7 days, continue with **A54** (Past Manic Episode), **page 22**. If criteria ultimately are not met for a Past Manic Episode, diagnose this episode as Other Specified Bipolar Disorder (**D23, page 51**).	— + ↓ Continue with **A53,** CRITERION F, **next page.**	A5

A53	IF UNKNOWN: **When did this period of being (high/irritable/OWN WORDS) begin?**	F. [Primary Hypomanic Episode] The episode is not attributable to the physiological effects of a substance (e.g., a drug of abuse, a medication, other treatment) or another medical condition.

Just before this began, were you physically ill?

   IF YES: **What did the doctor say?**

Just before this began, were you taking any medications?

   IF YES: **Any change in the amount you were taking?**

Just before this began, were you drinking or using any street drugs?

> Refer to the User's Guide, Section 9, for guidance on determining whether there is an etiological GMC or substance/medication.

Note: A full Hypomanic Episode that emerges during antidepressant treatment (e.g., medication, electroconvulsive therapy) but persists at a fully syndromal level beyond the physiological effect of that treatment is sufficient evidence for a Hypomanic Episode diagnosis. However, caution is indicated so that one or two symptoms (particularly increased irritability, edginess, or agitation following antidepressant use) are neither taken as sufficient for diagnosis of a Hypomanic Episode, nor necessarily indicative of a bipolar diathesis.

NOTE: Code "NO" only if episode _is_ due to a GMC or substance/medication.

Refer to list of etiological GMCs and substances/medications in **A40, page 19**.

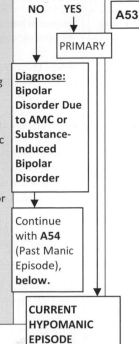

NO   YES   **A53**

PRIMARY

Diagnose: Bipolar Disorder Due to AMC or Substance-Induced Bipolar Disorder

Continue with A54 (Past Manic Episode), **below.**

CURRENT HYPOMANIC EPISODE Continue with **A54** (Past Manic Episode), **below.**

PAST MANIC EPISODE	**MANIC EPISODE CRITERIA**	
NOTE: IF THERE IS CURRENTLY ELEVATED OR IRRITABLE MOOD BUT FULL CRITERIA ARE NOT MET FOR A MANIC EPISODE, SUBSTITUTE THE PHRASE **"Has there ever been <u>another</u> time..."** *IN THE SCREENING QUESTIONS BELOW.*		

A54   **Have you <u>ever</u> had a period of time when you were feeling so good, "high," excited, or "on top of the world" that other people thought you were not your normal self?**

  ▶IF YES: **What was it like? (Was that more than just feeling good?)**

    Did you also feel like you were "hyper" or "wired" and had an unusual amount of energy? Were you much more active than is typical for you? (Did other people comment on how much you were doing?)

▶IF NO: **Have you <u>ever</u> had a period of time when you were feeling irritable, angry, or short-tempered for most of the day, for at least several days? (Was that different from the way you usually are?)** **What was it like?** **Did you also feel like you were "hyper" or "wired" and had an unusual amount of energy? Were you much more active than is typical for you? (Did other people comment on how much you were doing?)**	A. A distinct period [lasting at least several days] of abnormally and persistently elevated, expansive, or irritable mood and abnormally and persistently increased activity or energy.	— + **A54** Continue with **A78** (Persistent Depressive Disorder), **page 29.**

A55	Have you had more than one time like that? (Which time was the most intense or caused the most problems?)
	
	IF UNCLEAR: **Have you had any times like that since (ONE YEAR AGO)?**
	
	How long did this last? (As long as 1 week?)
	
	    IF LESS THAN ONE WEEK: **Did you need to go into the hospital to protect you from hurting yourself or someone else, or from doing something that could have caused serious financial or legal problems?**
	
	Did you feel (high/irritable/OWN WORDS) for most of the day, <u>nearly every day,</u> during this time?
		NOTE: If there is evidence for more than one past episode, select the one with the most impairment for your inquiry about past Manic Episode. If there was an episode in the past year, ask about that episode. If possible, avoid episodes that are likely to be substance-induced.
		
		...lasting at least 1 week and present most of the day, nearly every day (or any duration if hospitalization is necessary).
		
		*NOTE: IF ELEVATED MOOD LASTED LESS THAN 1 WEEK, CHECK WHETHER THERE HAS BEEN A PERIOD OF IRRITABLE MOOD LASTING AT LEAST 1 WEEK BEFORE SKIPPING TO **A66**.*
			— +
			    ↓
			Continue with **A66** (Past Hypomanic Episode), **page 26.**
				A5

	FOR **A56–A62**, FOCUS ON THE MOST SEVERE PERIOD OF THE EPISODE THAT YOU ARE INQUIRING ABOUT. IF UNKNOWN: **During (EPISODE), when were you the most (high/irritable/OWN WORDS)?**	B. During the period of mood disturbance and increased energy or activity, three (or more) of the following symptoms (four if the mood is only irritable) are present to a significant degree and represent a noticeable change from usual behavior:		
A56	During that time... **...how did you feel about yourself? (More self-confident than usual? Did you feel much smarter or better than everyone else? Did you feel like you had any special powers or abilities?)**	1. Inflated self-esteem or grandiosity.	— +	A5
A57	**...did you need less sleep than usual? (How much sleep did you get?)** IF YES: **Did you still feel rested?**	2. Decreased need for sleep (e.g., feels rested after only 3 hours of sleep).	— +	A5
A58	**...were you much more talkative than usual? (Did people have trouble stopping you or understanding you? Did people have trouble getting a word in edgewise?)**	3. More talkative than usual or pressure to keep talking.	— +	A5
A59	**...were your thoughts racing through your head? (What was that like?)**	4. Flight of ideas or subjective experience that thoughts are racing.	— +	A5
A60	**...were you so easily distracted by things around you that you had trouble concentrating or staying on one track? (Give me an example of that.)**	5. Distractibility (i.e., attention too easily drawn to unimportant or irrelevant external stimuli), as reported or observed.	— +	A6

A61	...how did you spend your time? (Work, friends, hobbies? Were you especially busy during that time?) (Did you find yourself more enthusiastic at work or working harder at your job? Did you find yourself more engaged in school activities or studying harder?) (Were you more sociable during that time, such as calling on friends or going out with them more than you usually do or making a lot of new friends?) (Were you spending more time thinking about sex or involved in doing something sexual, by yourself or with others? Was that a big change for you?) Were you physically restless during this time, doing things like pacing a lot, or being unable to sit still? (How bad was it?)	6. Increase in goal-directed activity (either socially, at work or school, or sexually) or psychomotor agitation (i.e., purposeless non-goal-directed activity).	—	+	A61
A62	...did you do anything that could have caused trouble for you or your family? (Spending money on things you didn't need or couldn't afford? How about giving away money or valuable things? Gambling with money you couldn't afford to lose?) (Anything sexual that was likely to get you in trouble? Driving recklessly?) (Did you make any risky or impulsive business investments or get involved in a business scheme that you wouldn't normally have done?)	7. Excessive involvement in activities that have a high potential for painful consequences (e.g., engaging in unrestrained buying sprees, sexual indiscretions, or foolish business investments).	—	+	A62
A63		AT LEAST THREE OF THE ABOVE CRITERION B SXS (A56–A62) ARE RATED "+" (FOUR IF MOOD ONLY IRRITABLE).	NO	YES	A63

IF NOT ALREADY ASKED: **Has there been any other time when you were (high/irritable/OWN WORDS) and had even more of the symptoms that I just asked you about?**

    IF YES: Go back to **A54, page 22,** and ask about that episode.

    IF NO: Continue with **A78** (Persistent Depressive Disorder), **page 29.**

Continue with **A64** (Criterion C), **next page.**

A64

IF UNCLEAR: **What effect did** (MANIC SXS) **have on your life?**

IF UNKNOWN: **Did you need to go into the hospital to protect you from hurting yourself or someone else, or from doing something that could have caused serious financial or legal problems?**

ASK THE FOLLOWING QUESTIONS <u>ONLY AS NEEDED</u>:

How did (MANIC SXS) **affect your relationships or your interactions with other people? (Did** [MANIC SXS] **cause you any problems in your relationships with your family, romantic partner, or friends?)**

How did (MANIC SXS) **affect your work/school? (How about your attendance at work/school? Did** [MANIC SXS] **make it more difficult to do your work/schoolwork)? Did** [MANIC SXS] **affect the quality of your work/schoolwork?)**

How did (MANIC SXS) **affect your ability to take care of things at home?**

C. The mood disturbance is sufficiently severe to cause marked impairment in social or occupational functioning or to necessitate hospitalization to prevent harm to self or others, or there are psychotic features.

—   +   **A6**

Continue with **A65**, below.

IF NOT ALREADY ASKED: **Has there been any other time when you were (high/irritable/OWN WORDS) and had** (ACKNOWLEDGED MANIC SXS) **and you got into trouble with people or were hospitalized?**

▶ IF YES: Go back to **A54**, **page 22**, and ask about that episode.

▶ IF NO: Go to **A78** (Persistent Depressive Disorder), **page 29**.

A65

IF UNKNOWN: **When did this period of being (high/irritable/OWN WORDS) begin?**

Just before this began, were you physically ill?

   IF YES: **What did the doctor say?**

Just before this began, were you taking any medications?

   IF YES: **Any change in the amount you were taking?**

Just before this began, were you drinking or using any street drugs?

┄┄┄┄┄┄┄┄┄┄┄┄┄┄┄┄┄┄┄┄┄┄┄┄┄
Refer to the User's Guide, Section 9, for guidance on determining whether there is an etiological GMC or substance/medication.
┄┄┄┄┄┄┄┄┄┄┄┄┄┄┄┄┄┄┄┄┄┄┄┄┄

D. [Primary Manic Episode] The episode is not attributable to the physiological effects of a substance (e.g., a drug of abuse, a medication, other treatment) or another medical condition.

Note: A full Manic Episode that emerges during antidepressant treatment (e.g., medication, electroconvulsive therapy) but persists at a fully syndromal level beyond the physiological effect of that treatment is sufficient evidence for a Manic Episode and, therefore, a Bipolar I [Disorder] diagnosis.

NOTE: Code "NO" only if episode is due to a GMC or substance/medication.

*Refer to list of etiological GMCs and substances/medications in **A40, page 19**.*

NO   YES   **A6**

PRIMARY

Diagnose: **Bipolar Disorder Due to AMC or Substance-Induced Bipolar Disorder**

PAST MANIC EPISODE Continue with **B1** (Psychotic Symptoms), **page 31**.

Has there been any other time when you were (high/irritable/OWN WORDS) and had (ACKNOWLEDGED MANIC SXS) **and you were not (ill with GMC/using SUBSTANCE)?**

▶ IF YES: Go back to **A54**, **page 22**, and ask about that episode.

▶ IF NO: Continue with **A78** (Persistent Depressive Disorder), **page 29**.

	PAST HYPOMANIC EPISODE	HYPOMANIC EPISODE CRITERIA		
A66	IF UNKNOWN: **Have you had more than one time like that?** IF YES: **Which time was the most intense or extreme?** IF UNCLEAR: **Have you had any times like that in the last year, since** (ONE YEAR AGO)**?** **Did that period when you were (high/irritable/OWN WORDS) last for at least 4 days?** <u>**Was it for most of the day, nearly every day?**</u>	A. A distinct period of abnormally and persistently elevated, expansive, or irritable mood and abnormally and persistently increased activity or energy, lasting at least 4 consecutive days and present most of the day, nearly every day. *NOTE: If there is evidence for more than one past episode, select the "worst" (most intense) one for your inquiry about past Hypomanic Episode. If there was an episode in the past year, ask about that episode. If possible, avoid episodes that are likely to be substance-induced.*	— ↓ + Continue with **A78** (Persistent Depressive Disorder), **page 29.**	**A66**
		B. During the period of mood disturbance and increased energy and activity, three (or more) of the following symptoms (four if the mood is only irritable) have persisted, represent a noticeable change from usual behavior, and have been present to a significant degree:		
A67	**During that time...** **...how did you feel about yourself? (More self-confident than usual? Did you feel much smarter or better than everyone else? Did you feel like you had any special powers or abilities?)**	1. Inflated self-esteem or grandiosity.	— +	**A67**
A68	**...did you need less sleep than usual? (How much sleep did you get?)** IF YES: **Did you still feel rested?**	2. Decreased need for sleep (e.g., feels rested after only 3 hours of sleep).	— +	**A68**
A69	**...were you much more talkative than usual? (Did people have trouble stopping you or understanding you? Did people have trouble getting a word in edgewise?)**	3. More talkative than usual or pressure to keep talking.	— +	**A69**
A70	**...were your thoughts racing through your head? (What was that like?)**	4. Flight of ideas or subjective experience that thoughts are racing.	— +	**A70**
A71	**...were you so easily distracted by things around you that you had trouble concentrating or staying on one track? (Give me an example of that.)**	5. Distractibility (i.e., attention too easily drawn to unimportant or irrelevant external stimuli), as reported or observed.	— +	**A71**

A72	...how did you spend your time? (Work, friends, hobbies? Were you especially productive or busy during that time?) (Did you find yourself more enthusiastic at work or working harder at your job? Did you find yourself more engaged in school activities or studying harder?) (Were you more sociable during that time, such as calling on friends or going out with them more than you usually do or making a lot of new friends?) (Were you spending more time thinking about sex or involved in doing something sexual, by yourself or with others? Was that a big change for you?) Were you physically restless during this time, doing things like pacing a lot, or being unable to sit still? (How bad was it?)	6. Increase in goal-directed activity (either socially, at work or school, or sexually) or psychomotor agitation.	—	+	A7
A73	...did you do anything that could have caused trouble for you or your family? (Spending money on things you didn't need or couldn't afford? How about giving away money or valuable things? Gambling with money you couldn't afford to lose?) (Anything sexual that was likely to get you in trouble? Driving recklessly?) (Did you make any risky or impulsive business investments or get involved in a business scheme that you wouldn't normally have done?)	7. Excessive involvement in activities that have a high potential for painful consequences (e.g., engaging in unrestrained buying sprees, sexual indiscretions, or foolish business investments).	—	+	A7
A73a		AT LEAST THREE OF THE ABOVE CRITERION B SXS **(A67–A73)** ARE RATED "+" (FOUR IF MOOD ONLY IRRITABLE).	**NO**	**YES**	A7:

IF NOT ALREADY ASKED: **Has there been any other time when you were (high/irritable/OWN WORDS) and had even more of the symptoms that I just asked you about?**

> IF YES: Go back to **A66**, **page 26**, and ask about that episode.
>
> IF NO: Continue with **A78** (Persistent Depressive Disorder), **page 29.**

Continue with **A74,** (Criterion C), **below.**

A74	IF UNCLEAR: **Was this very different from the way you usually are when you are not (high/irritable/OWN WORDS)? (How were you different? At work? With friends?)**	C. The episode is associated with an unequivocal change in functioning that is uncharacteristic of the individual when not symptomatic.	—	+	A7

IF NOT ALREADY ASKED: **Has there been any other time when you were (high/irritable/OWN WORDS) in which you were really different from the way you usually are?**

> IF YES: Go back to **A66**, **page 26**, and ask about that episode.
>
> IF NO: Continue with **A78** (Persistent Depressive Disorder), **page 29.**

Continue with **A75** (Criterion D), **next page.**

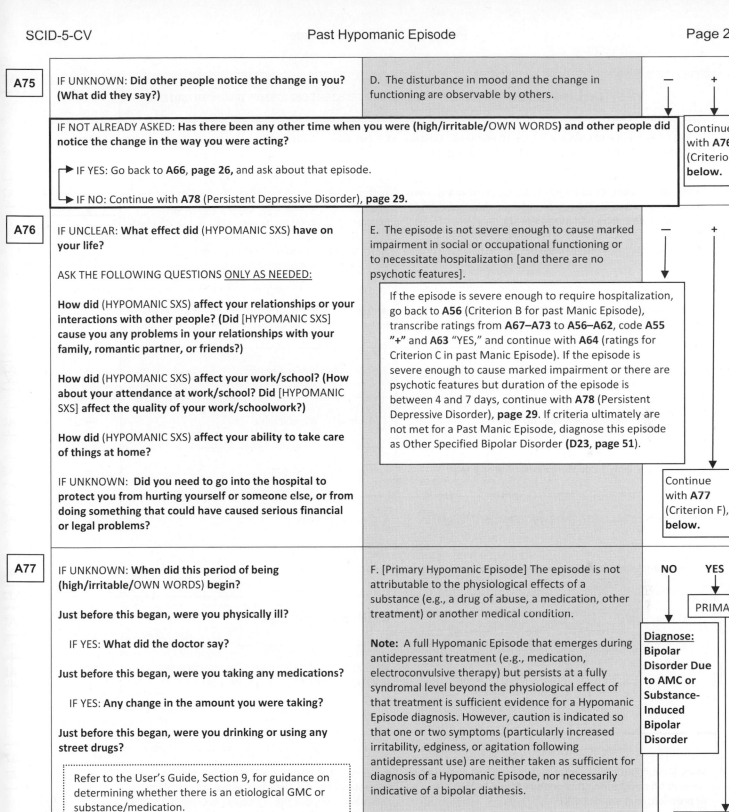

A75

IF UNKNOWN: **Did other people notice the change in you? (What did they say?)**

D. The disturbance in mood and the change in functioning are observable by others.

—   +

A75

Continue with **A76** (Criterion E), **below.**

IF NOT ALREADY ASKED: **Has there been any other time when you were (high/irritable/OWN WORDS) and other people did notice the change in the way you were acting?**

➤ IF YES: Go back to **A66**, **page 26,** and ask about that episode.

➤ IF NO: Continue with **A78** (Persistent Depressive Disorder), **page 29.**

A76

IF UNCLEAR: **What effect did** (HYPOMANIC SXS) **have on your life?**

ASK THE FOLLOWING QUESTIONS ONLY AS NEEDED:

How did (HYPOMANIC SXS) **affect your relationships or your interactions with other people? (Did [HYPOMANIC SXS] cause you any problems in your relationships with your family, romantic partner, or friends?)**

How did (HYPOMANIC SXS) **affect your work/school? (How about your attendance at work/school? Did [HYPOMANIC SXS] affect the quality of your work/schoolwork?)**

How did (HYPOMANIC SXS) **affect your ability to take care of things at home?**

IF UNKNOWN: **Did you need to go into the hospital to protect you from hurting yourself or someone else, or from doing something that could have caused serious financial or legal problems?**

E. The episode is not severe enough to cause marked impairment in social or occupational functioning or to necessitate hospitalization [and there are no psychotic features].

If the episode is severe enough to require hospitalization, go back to **A56** (Criterion B for past Manic Episode), transcribe ratings from **A67–A73** to **A56–A62,** code **A55** "**+**" and **A63** "YES," and continue with **A64** (ratings for Criterion C in past Manic Episode). If the episode is severe enough to cause marked impairment or there are psychotic features but duration of the episode is between 4 and 7 days, continue with **A78** (Persistent Depressive Disorder), **page 29.** If criteria ultimately are not met for a Past Manic Episode, diagnose this episode as Other Specified Bipolar Disorder (**D23, page 51**).

—   +

A76

Continue with **A77** (Criterion F), **below.**

A77

IF UNKNOWN: **When did this period of being (high/irritable/OWN WORDS) begin?**

Just before this began, were you physically ill?

IF YES: **What did the doctor say?**

Just before this began, were you taking any medications?

IF YES: **Any change in the amount you were taking?**

Just before this began, were you drinking or using any street drugs?

Refer to the User's Guide, Section 9, for guidance on determining whether there is an etiological GMC or substance/medication.

F. [Primary Hypomanic Episode] The episode is not attributable to the physiological effects of a substance (e.g., a drug of abuse, a medication, other treatment) or another medical condition.

Note: A full Hypomanic Episode that emerges during antidepressant treatment (e.g., medication, electroconvulsive therapy) but persists at a fully syndromal level beyond the physiological effect of that treatment is sufficient evidence for a Hypomanic Episode diagnosis. However, caution is indicated so that one or two symptoms (particularly increased irritability, edginess, or agitation following antidepressant use) are neither taken as sufficient for diagnosis of a Hypomanic Episode, nor necessarily indicative of a bipolar diathesis.

NOTE: Code "NO" only if episode is due to a GMC or substance/medication.

Refer to list of etiological GMCs and substances/medications in ***A40, page 19.***

NO   YES

A77

PRIMARY

Diagnose: **Bipolar Disorder Due to AMC or Substance-Induced Bipolar Disorder**

PAST HYPOMANIC EPISODE Continue with **B1** (Psychotic Symptoms), **page 31.**

IF NOT ALREADY ASKED: **Has there been any other time when you were (high/irritable/OWN WORDS) and had (ACKNOWLEDGED HYPOMANIC SXS) and you were not (ill with GMC/using SUBSTANCE)?**

➤ IF YES: Go back to **A66**, **page 26,** and ask about that episode.

➤ IF NO: Continue with **A78** (Persistent Depressive Disorder), **page 29.**

	PERSISTENT DEPRESSIVE DISORDER	PERSISTENT DEPRESSIVE DISORDER CRITERIA		
	IF: THERE HAS EVER BEEN A MANIC OR HYPOMANIC EPISODE, SKIP THE ASSESSMENT OF PERSISTENT DEPRESSIVE DISORDER AND CONTINUE WITH **B1** (PSYCHOTIC SYMPTOMS), **PAGE 31**.			
A78	In the past 2 years, since (TWO YEARS AGO), **have you been bothered by depressed mood most of the day, more days than not? (More than half of the time?)** IF YES: **What has that been like?**	A. Depressed mood for most of the day, for more days than not, as indicated either by subjective account or observation by others, for at least 2 years. **Note:** In children and adolescents, mood can be irritable and duration must be at least 1 year.	— + ↓ Continue with **B1** (Psychotic Symptoms), **page 31**.	A7
	During these periods of (OWN WORDS FOR CHRONIC DEPRESSION) **did you often...**	B. Presence, while depressed, of two (or more) of the following:		
A79	**...lose your appetite? (What about overeating?)**	1. Poor appetite or overeating.	— +	A7
A80	**...have trouble sleeping or sleep too much?**	2. Insomnia or hypersomnia.	— +	A8
A81	**...have little energy to do things or feel tired a lot?**	3. Low energy or fatigue.	— +	A8
A82	**...feel down on yourself? (Feel worthless, or a failure?)**	4. Low self-esteem.	— +	A8
A83	**...have trouble concentrating or making decisions?**	5. Poor concentration or difficulty making decisions.	— +	A8
A84	**...feel hopeless?**	6. Feelings of hopelessness.	— +	A8
A85		AT LEAST TWO OF THE ABOVE CRITERION B SXS (A79–A84) ARE RATED "+".	NO YES ↓ Continue with **B1** (Psychotic Symptoms), **page 31**.	A8
A86	**Since** (TWO YEARS AGO), **what was the longest period of time up till now, during this period of long-lasting depression, that you felt OK?**	C. During the 2-year period (1 year for children or adolescents) of the disturbance, the individual has never been without the symptoms in Criteria A and B for more than 2 months at a time. *NOTE: CRITERION D HAS BEEN INTENTIONALLY OMITTED.*	— + ↓ Continue with **B1** (Psychotic Symptoms), **page 31**.	A8
A87		E. There has never been a Manic Episode or a Hypomanic Episode, and criteria have never been met for Cyclothymic Disorder.	— + ↓ Continue with **B1** (Psychotic Symptoms), **page 31**.	A8

| A88 | IF NOT ALREADY CLEAR: RETURN TO THIS ITEM AFTER COMPLETING THE PSYCHOTIC DISORDERS SECTION. | F. The disturbance is not better explained by a persistent Schizoaffective Disorder, Schizophrenia, Delusional Disorder, or Other Specified or Unspecified Schizophrenia Spectrum and Other Psychotic Disorder.

NOTE: CODE "+" IF NO PERSISTENT PSYCHOTIC DISORDER OR IF NOT BETTER EXPLAINED BY A PERSISTENT PSYCHOTIC DISORDER. | —   +
↓
Continue with **B1** (Psychotic Symptoms), **page 31.** | A88 |

| A89 | IF UNKNOWN; **When did this begin?**

Just before this began, were you physically ill?

   IF YES: **What did the doctor say?**

Just before this began, were you taking any medications?

   IF YES: **Any change in the amount you were taking?**

Just before this began, were you drinking or using any street drugs?

Refer to the User's Guide, Section 9, for guidance on determining whether there is an etiological GMC or substance/medication. | G. [Primary Depressive Disorder] The symptoms are not attributable to the physiological effects of a substance (e.g., a drug of abuse, a medication) or another medical condition (e.g., hypothyroidism).

*Refer to list of etiological GMCs and substances/medications in **A12, page 12.*** | NO   YES
         PRIMARY

Diagnose: Depressive Disorder Due to AMC or Substance-Induced Depressive Disorder

Continue with **B1** (Psychotic Symptoms), **page 31.**   Continue with **A90, below.** | A89 |

| A90 | IF UNCLEAR: **What effect have** (DEPRESSIVE SXS) **had on your life?**

ASK THE FOLLOWING QUESTIONS <u>ONLY AS NEEDED</u>:

How have (DEPRESSIVE SXS) **affected your relationships or your interactions with other people? (Have** [DEPRESSIVE SXS] **caused you any problems in your relationships with your family, romantic partner, or friends?)**

How have (DEPRESSIVE SXS) **affected your work/school? (How about your attendance at work/school? Have** [DEPRESSIVE SXS] **made it more difficult to do your work/schoolwork? Have** [DEPRESSIVE SXS] **affected the quality of your work/schoolwork?)**

How have (DEPRESSIVE SXS) **affected your ability to take care of things at home? How about doing simple everyday things, like getting dressed, bathing, or brushing your teeth? How about doing other things that are important to you, like religious activities, physical exercise, or hobbies? Did you avoid doing anything because you felt like you weren't up to it?**

Have (DEPRESSIVE SXS) **affected any other important part of your life?**

IF DOES NOT INTERFERE WITH LIFE: **How much have you been bothered or upset by having** (DEPRESSIVE SXS)**?** | H. The symptoms cause clinically significant distress or impairment in social, occupational, or other important areas of functioning. | —   +
↓
Continue with **B1** (Psychotic Symptoms), **page 31.**

Diagnose: Persistent Depressive Disorder (current). Continue with **B1** (Psychotic Symptoms), **page 31.** | A90 |

B. PSYCHOTIC AND ASSOCIATED SYMPTOMS

FOR ANY PSYCHOTIC AND ASSOCIATED SYMPTOMS THAT ARE PRESENT, DETERMINE WHETHER THE SYMPTOM IS DEFINITELY "PRIMARY" (I.E., DUE TO A PSYCHOTIC DISORDER) OR WHETHER THERE IS A POSSIBLE OR DEFINITE ETIOLOGICAL GMC OR SUBSTANCE/MEDICATION. (REFER TO **C6, PAGE 38,** FOR A LIST OF ETIOLOGICAL GMCs OR SUBSTANCES/MEDICATIONS.) THIS INFORMATION WILL BE USEFUL IN DIFFERENTIATING A PRIMARY PSYCHOTIC DISORDER FROM A PSYCHOTIC DISORDER DUE TO AMC OR SUBSTANCE/MEDICATION-INDUCED PSYCHOTIC DISORDER IN MODULE C.

THE FOLLOWING QUESTIONS MAY BE USEFUL FOR THIS DETERMINATION IF THE OVERVIEW HAS NOT ALREADY PROVIDED THE INFORMATION:

Just before (PSYCHOTIC SXS) **began, were you using drugs?** IF YES: **What were you using?**
...On any medications? IF YES: **What were you taking?**
...Did you drink much more than usual or stop drinking after you had been drinking a lot for a while?
...Were you physically ill?

IF YES TO ANY: **Has there been a time when you had** (PSYCHOTIC SXS) **and were not (using** [DRUG]**/taking** [MEDICATION]**/changing your drinking habits/physically ill)?**

Now I am going to ask you about unusual experiences that people sometimes have.

DELUSIONS

A false belief based on incorrect inference about external reality that is firmly held despite what almost everyone else believes and despite what constitutes incontrovertible and obvious proof or evidence to the contrary. The belief is not one ordinarily accepted by other members of the person's culture or subculture (i.e., it is not an article of religious faith). When a false belief involves a value judgment, it is regarded as a delusion only when the judgment is so extreme as to defy credibility.

NOTE: Code overvalued ideas (unreasonable and sustained beliefs that are maintained with less than delusional intensity) as "—".

| B1 | Has it ever seemed like people were talking about you or taking special notice of you? (What do you think they were saying about you?)

IF YES: Were you convinced they were talking about you or did you think it might have been your imagination?

Did you ever have the feeling that something on the radio, TV, or in a movie was meant especially for you? (Not just that it was particularly relevant to you, but that it was specifically meant for you.)

Did you ever have the feeling that the words in a popular song were meant to send you a special message?

Did you ever have the feeling that what people were wearing was intended to send you a special message?

Did you ever have the feeling that street signs or billboards had a special meaning for you? | **Delusion of reference** (i.e., a belief that events, objects, or other people in the individual's immediate environment have a particular or unusual significance)

DESCRIBE: | — + | B1 |
| B2 | What about anyone going out of their way to give you a hard time, or trying to hurt you? (Tell me about that.)

Have you ever had the feeling that you were being followed, spied on, manipulated, or plotted against?

Did you ever have the feeling that you were being poisoned or that your food had been tampered with? | **Persecutory delusion** (i.e., a belief that the individual [or his or her group] is being attacked, harassed, cheated, persecuted, or conspired against)

DESCRIBE: | — + | B2 |

B3	Have you ever thought that you were especially important in some way, or that you had special powers or knowledge? (Tell me about that.) Did you ever believe that you had a special or close relationship with a celebrity or someone else famous?	**Grandiose delusion** (i.e., content involves exaggerated power, knowledge or importance, or a special relationship to a deity or famous person) DESCRIBE:	—	+	B3
B4	Have you ever been convinced that something was very wrong with your physical health even though your doctor said nothing was wrong...like you had cancer or some other disease? (Tell me about that.) Have you ever felt that something strange was happening to parts of your body?	**Somatic delusion** (i.e., content involves change or disturbance in body appearance or functioning) DESCRIBE:	—	+	B4
B5	Have you ever felt that you had committed a crime or done something terrible for which you should be punished? (Tell me about that.) Have you ever felt that something you did, or should have done but did not do, caused serious harm to your parents, children, other family members, or friends? (Tell me about that.) What about feeling responsible for a disaster such as a fire, flood, or earthquake? (Tell me about that.)	**Delusion of guilt** (i.e., a belief that a minor error in the past will lead to disaster, or that he or she has committed a horrible crime and should be punished severely, or that he or she is responsible for a disaster [e.g., an earthquake or fire] with which there can be no possible connection) DESCRIBE:	—	+	B5
B6	Have you ever been convinced that your spouse or partner was being unfaithful to you? IF YES: How did you know he/she was being unfaithful? (What clued you into this?)	**Jealous delusion** (i.e., a belief that one's sexual partner is unfaithful) DESCRIBE:	—	+	B6
B7	Are you a religious or spiritual person? ▶IF YES: Have you ever had any religious or spiritual experiences that the other people in your religious or spiritual community have not experienced? ▶IF YES: Tell me about your experiences. (What did they think about these experiences of yours?) ▶IF NO: Have you ever felt that God, the devil, or some other spiritual being or higher power has communicated directly with you? (Tell me about that. Do others in your religious or spiritual community also have such experiences?) ▶ IF NO: Have you ever felt that God, or the devil or some other spiritual being or higher power has communicated directly with you? (Tell me about that. Do others in your religious or spiritual community also have such experiences?)	**Religious delusion** (i.e., a delusion with a religious or spiritual content) DESCRIBE:	—	+	B7

B8	Did you ever have a "secret admirer" who, when you tried to contact them, denied that they were in love with you? (Tell me about that.) Were you ever romantically involved with someone famous? (Tell me about that.)	**Erotomanic delusion** (i.e., a belief that another person, usually of higher status, is in love with the individual) DESCRIBE:	— +	B8
B9	Did you ever feel that someone or something outside yourself was controlling your thoughts or actions against your will? (Tell me about that.)	**Delusion of being controlled** (i.e., feelings, impulses, thoughts, or actions are experienced as being under the control of some external force rather than under one's own control) DESCRIBE:	— +	B9
B10	Did you ever feel that certain thoughts that were not your own were put into your head? (Tell me about that.)	**Thought insertion** (i.e., a belief that certain thoughts are not one's own, but rather are inserted into one's mind) DESCRIBE:	— +	B1
B11	What about thoughts being taken out of your head? (Tell me about that.)	**Thought withdrawal** (i.e., a belief that one's thoughts have been "removed" by some outside force) DESCRIBE:	— +	B1
B12	Did you ever feel as if your thoughts were being broadcast out loud so that other people could actually hear what you were thinking? (Tell me about that.)	**Thought broadcasting** (i.e., a delusion that one's thoughts are being broadcast out loud so that others can perceive them) DESCRIBE:	— +	B1
B13	Did you ever believe that someone could read your mind? (Tell me about that.)	**Other delusions** (e.g., a belief that others can read the person's mind, a delusion that one has died several years ago) DESCRIBE:	— +	B1

HALLUCINATIONS

A perception-like experience with the clarity and impact of a true perception, but without the external stimulation of the relevant sensory organ. The person may or may not have insight into the nonveridical nature of the hallucination (i.e., one hallucinating person may recognize the false sensory experience, whereas another may be convinced that the experience is grounded in reality).

NOTE: Code "—" for hallucinations that are so transient as to be without diagnostic significance.
Code "—" for hypnagogic or hynopompic hallucinations occurring only when falling asleep or upon awakening, respectively.

B14	Did you ever hear things that other people couldn't, such as noises, or the voices of people whispering or talking? (Were you awake at the time?) IF YES: **What did you hear? How often did you hear it?**	**Auditory hallucinations** (i.e., a hallucination involving the perception of sound, most commonly of voice, when fully awake, heard either inside or outside of one's head) DESCRIBE:	— +	B1

B15	Did you have visions or see things that other people couldn't see? (Tell me about that. Were you awake at the time?)	**Visual hallucinations** (i.e., a hallucination involving sight, which may consist of formed images, such as of people, or of unformed images, such as flashes of light) *NOTE: Distinguish from an illusion (i.e., a misperception of a real external stimulus).* DESCRIBE:	− +	**B15**
B16	What about strange sensations on your skin, like feeling like something is creeping or crawling on or under your skin? How about the feeling of being touched or stroked? (Tell me about that.)	**Tactile hallucinations** (i.e., a hallucination involving the perception of being touched or of something being under one's skin) DESCRIBE	− +	**B16**
B17	What about having unusual sensations inside a part of your body, like a feeling of electricity? (Tell me about that.)	**Somatic hallucinations** (i.e., a hallucination involving the perception of physical experience localized within the body [e.g., a feeling of electricity]) DESCRIBE:	− +	**B17**
B18	How about eating or drinking something that you thought tasted bad or strange even though everyone else who tasted it thought it was fine? (Tell me about that.)	**Gustatory hallucinations** (i.e., a hallucination involving the perception of taste [usually unpleasant]) DESCRIBE:	− +	**B18**
B19	What about smelling unpleasant things that other people couldn't smell, like decaying food or dead bodies? (Tell me about that.)	**Olfactory hallucinations** (i.e., a hallucination involving the perception of odor) DESCRIBE:	− +	**B19**

DISORGANIZED SPEECH AND BEHAVIOR AND CATATONIA

(Let me stop for a minute while I make a few notes...)

THE FOLLOWING ITEMS ARE RATED BASED ON OBSERVATION AND HISTORY (CONSULT OLD CHARTS, OTHER OBSERVERS— E.G., FAMILY MEMBERS, THERAPEUTIC STAFF)

B20		**DISORGANIZED SPEECH:** The individual may switch from one topic to another (derailment or loose associations). Answers to questions may be obliquely related or completely unrelated (tangentiality). Rarely, speech may be so severely disorganized that it is nearly incomprehensible and resembles receptive aphasia in its linguistic disorganization (incoherence or "word salad"). Because mildly disorganized speech is common and nonspecific, the symptom must be severe enough to substantially impair effective communication. DESCRIBE:	− +	**B20**

B21		**GROSSLY DISORGANIZED BEHAVIOR:** May range from childlike silliness to unpredictable agitation. The person may appear markedly disheveled, may dress in an unusual manner (e.g., wearing multiple overcoats, scarves, and gloves on a hot day), or may display clearly inappropriate sexual behavior (e.g., public masturbation) or unpredictable and untriggered agitation (e.g., shouting or swearing). DESCRIBE:	— + **B2**

B22	THE FOLLOWING SIX ITEMS CAN BE ASSESSED BY **OBSERVATION** OR BY REPORTS OF INFORMANTS (CONSULT PATIENT RECORDS, OTHER OBSERVERS SUCH AS FAMILY MEMBERS, THERAPEUTIC STAFF).	**CATATONIC BEHAVIOR** **Stupor** (i.e., no psychomotor activity; not actively relating to environment) **Grimacing** (i.e., odd and inappropriate facial expressions unrelated to situation) **Mannerism** (i.e., odd, circumstantial caricature of normal actions) **Posturing** (i.e., spontaneous and active maintenance of a posture against gravity) **Agitation, not influenced by external stimuli** **Stereotypy** (i.e., repetitive, abnormally frequent, non-goal-directed movements)	— + **B2**
	THE FOLLOWING THREE ITEMS CAN BE ASSESSED DURING THE **INTERVIEW** OR VIA INFORMANTS.	**Mutism** (i.e., no, or very little, verbal response [exclude if known aphasia]) **Echolalia** (i.e., mimicking another's speech) **Negativism** (i.e., opposition or no response to instructions or external stimuli)	
	THE FOLLOWING THREE ITEMS CAN BE ASSESSED DURING **PHYSICAL EXAMINATION** OR VIA INFORMANTS.	**Echopraxia** (i.e., mimicking another's movements) **Catalepsy** (i.e., passive induction of a posture held against gravity) **Waxy flexibility** (i.e., slight, even resistance to positioning by examiner) DESCRIBE:	

NEGATIVE SYMPTOMS

For any negative symptoms rated "+", determine whether the symptom is definitely primary (i.e., due to a Psychotic Disorder) or whether it is possibly or definitely secondary—i.e., related to another mental disorder (e.g., depression), a substance or a GMC (e.g., medication-induced akinesia), or a psychotic symptom (e.g., command hallucinations not to move).

B23	RATE THIS ITEM BASED ON INFORMATION OBTAINED FROM THE OVERVIEW. IF UNKNOWN: **Has there been a period of time lasting at least several months when you were not working, not in school, or doing much of anything?** IF UNKNOWN: **How about a period of time when you were unable to take care of basic everyday things, like brushing your teeth or bathing?** IF NO: **Did anyone ever say that you were not taking care of these or other basic everyday things?**	**Avolition:** An inability to initiate and persist in goal-directed activities. When severe enough to be considered pathological, avolition is pervasive and prevents the person from completing many different types of activities (e.g., work, intellectual pursuits, self-care).	− + ↓ − + POSSIBLY/ PRIMARY DEFINITELY SECONDARY	**B23**
B24		**Diminished Emotional Expressiveness:** Includes reductions in the expression of emotions in the face, eye contact, intonation of speech (prosody), and movements of the hand, head, and face that normally give an emotional emphasis to speech.	− + ↓ − + POSSIBLY/ PRIMARY DEFINITELY SECONDARY	**B24**

Continue with **C1** (Differential Diagnosis of Psychotic Disorders), **page 37.**

C. DIFFERENTIAL DIAGNOSIS OF PSYCHOTIC DISORDERS

If no psychotic items from Module B have ever been present, skip to **D1** (Differential Diagnosis of Mood Disorders), **page 45.**

When making the ratings for **C2, C3, C5, C6, C8, C16, C17,** and **C19-C21,** if it is not possible to determine whether a rating is "YES" or "NO," skip to **C22** (Other Specified Psychotic Disorder), **page 42.**

C1

Psychotic symptoms occur at times other than during Major Depressive **(A12/A26)** or Manic Episodes **(A40/A65).**

> *The following question may be asked for clarification:* IF A MAJOR DEPRESSIVE OR MANIC EPISODE HAS EVER BEEN PRESENT: **Has there ever been a time when you had** (PSYCHOTIC SXS) **and you were not (depressed/high/irritable/**OWN WORDS**)?**

YES

NO → Psychotic Mood Disorder
Go to **D1** (Differential Diagnosis of Mood Disorders), **page 45.**   **C1**

CRITERIA FOR SCHIZOPHRENIA
NOTE: Criteria are in a different order than in DSM-5.

C2

A. Two (or more) of the following, each present for a significant portion of time during a 1-month period (or less if successfully treated): At least one of these must be (1), (2), or (3):

1. Delusions **[B1–B13].**

2. Hallucinations **[B14–B19].**

3. Disorganized speech (e.g., frequent derailment or incoherence) **[B20].**

4. Grossly disorganized or catatonic behavior **[B21–B22].**

5. Negative symptoms (i.e., diminished emotional expression or avolition) **[B23–B24].**

NOTE: Consider rating "NO" if the only symptoms are delusions accompanied by tactile and/or olfactory hallucinations that are thematically related to the content of the delusions (which is consistent with a diagnosis of Delusional Disorder).

YES

NO → Go to **C13** (Delusional Disorder), **page 40.**   **C2**

C3

D. Schizoaffective Disorder and Depressive or Bipolar Disorder With Psychotic Features have been ruled out because either

1) No Major Depressive **[A12/A26]** or Manic Episodes **[A40/A65]** have occurred concurrently with the active-phase symptoms [i.e., Criterion A symptoms listed above in **C2**], or

> *The following question may be asked for clarification:* **Has there ever been a time when you had** (SXS FROM ACTIVE PHASE) **at the same time that you were (depressed/high/irritable/**OWN WORDS**)?**

2) If mood episodes have occurred during active-phase symptoms, they have been present for a minority [i.e., less than 50%] of the total duration of the active and residual periods of the illness.

> *The following question may be asked for clarification:* **How much of the time that you have had** (SXS FROM ACTIVE AND RESIDUAL PERIODS) **would you say you have also been (depressed/high/ irritable/**OWN WORDS**)?**

NOTE: Code "YES" if there have never been any Major Depressive or Manic Episodes OR if all episodes occurred during the prodromal or residual phase OR if mood episodes have been present for a minority of the total disturbance. Code "NO" only if mood episodes overlap with active-phase symptoms AND mood episodes have been present for a majority (50% or more) of the total duration of the illness.

YES

NO → Go to **C9** (Schizoaffective Disorder), **page 39.**   **C3**

C4

C. Continuous signs of the disturbance persist for at least 6 months. This 6-month period must include at least 1 month of symptoms (or less if successfully treated) that meet Criterion A (i.e., active-phase symptoms) and may include periods of prodromal or residual symptoms. During these prodromal or residual periods, the signs of the disturbance may be manifested by only negative symptoms [i.e., diminished emotional expression or avolition] or by two or more symptoms listed in Criterion A present in an attenuated form (e.g., odd beliefs, unusual perceptual experiences).

Prodromal/residual symptoms include:
- Unusual or odd beliefs that are not of delusional proportions (e.g., ideas of reference or magical thinking);
- Unusual perceptual experiences (e.g., sensing the presence of an unseen person);
- Speech that is generally understandable but digressive, vague, or overelaborate
- Behavior that is unusual but not grossly disorganized (e.g., collecting garbage, talking to self in public, hoarding food)
- Negative symptoms (e.g., marked impairment in personal hygiene and grooming; marked lack of initiative, interests, or energy)
- Blunted or inappropriate affect
- Marked social isolation or withdrawal

YES ↓

NO → Go to **C7** (Schizophreniform Disorder), **page 39.** **C4**

C5

B. For a significant portion of the time since the onset of the disturbance, level of functioning in one or more major areas, such as work, interpersonal relations, or self-care, is markedly below the level achieved prior to the onset (or when the onset is in childhood or adolescence, there is failure to achieve expected level of interpersonal, academic, or occupational functioning).

> *The following question may be asked for clarification:* **Since you got sick, was there a period of time when you had a lot of difficulty functioning? (Like being unable to work or go to school or not being able to take care of yourself? How about having difficulties with family members or friends, or not wanting to be around other people?)**

YES ↓

NO → Go to **C22** (Other Specified Psychotic Disorder), **page 42.** **C5**

C6

E. [Primary Psychotic Disorder] The disturbance is not attributable to the physiological effects of a substance (e.g., a drug of abuse, a medication) or another medical condition.

> *The following question may be asked for clarification:* **Just before this began, were you physically ill? Just before this began, were you taking any medications? Just before this began, were you using any street drugs?**

....
Refer to the User's Guide, Section 9, for guidance on determining whether there is an etiological GMC or substance/medication.
....

Etiological GMCs include neurological conditions (e.g., neoplasms, cerebrovascular disease, Huntington's disease, multiple sclerosis, epilepsy, auditory or visual nerve injury or impairment, deafness, migraine, central nervous system infections), endocrine conditions (e.g., hyper- and hypothyroidism, hyper- and hypoparathyroidism, hyper- and hypoadrenocorticism), metabolic conditions (e.g., hypoxia, hypercarbia, hypoglycemia), fluid or electrolyte imbalances, hepatic or renal diseases, and autoimmune disorders with central nervous system involvement (e.g., systemic lupus erythematosus).

Etiological substances/medications include alcohol (I/W); cannabis (I); hallucinogens (I), phencyclidine and related substances (I); inhalants (I); sedatives, hypnotics, and anxiolytics (I/W); stimulants (including cocaine) (I); anesthetics and analgesics; anticholinergic agents; anticonvulsants; antihistamines; antihypertensive and cardiovascular medications; antimicrobial medications; antiparkinsonian medications; chemotherapeutic agents (e.g., cyclosporine, procarbazine); corticosteroids; gastrointestinal medications; muscle relaxants; nonsteroidal anti-inflammatory medications; other over-the-counter medications (e.g., phenylephrine, pseudoephedrine); antidepressant medication; and disulfiram. Toxins include anticholinesterase, organophosphate insecticides, sarin and other nerve gases, carbon monoxide, carbon dioxide, and volatile substances such as fuel or paint.

YES (not due to a GMC or substance/medication) ↓

NO → **Diagnose: Psychotic Disorder Due to AMC or Substance-Induced Psychotic Disorder.** Go back to **C2, page 37,** if there are other psychotic symptoms not due to a GMC or substance/medication. Otherwise, go to **D1** (Differential Diagnosis of Mood Disorders), **page 45.** **C6**

SCHIZOPHRENIA
Go to **C25** (Chronology of Psychotic Disorders), **page 44.**

CRITERIA FOR SCHIZOPHRENIFORM DISORDER

C7

B. [Symptoms meeting Criterion A of Schizophrenia **(C2)** last] at least 1 month but less than 6 months.

> *The following question may be asked for clarification:* **How long did** (PSYCHOTIC SXS) **last?**

YES

NO → Go to **C19** (Brief Psychotic Disorder), **page 41.** **C7**

C8

D. [Primary Psychotic Disorder] The disturbance is not attributable to the physiological effects of a substance (e.g., a drug of abuse, a medication) or another medical condition.

> *The following question may be asked for clarification:* **Just before this began, were you physically ill? Just before this began, were you taking any medications? Just before this began, were you using any street drugs?**

*Refer to list of etiological GMCs and substances/medications in **C6, page 38.***

> Refer to the User's Guide, Section 9, for guidance on determining whether there is an etiological GMC or substance/medication.

YES (not due to a GMC or substance/medication)

> **SCHIZOPHRENIFORM DISORDER**
> Go to **C26** (Chronology), **page 44.**

NO

Diagnose: Psychotic Disorder Due to AMC or Substance-Induced Psychotic Disorder. Go back to **C2, page 37,** if there are other psychotic symptoms not due to a GMC or substance/medication. Otherwise, go to **D1** (Differential Diagnosis of Mood Disorders), **page 45.** **C8**

CRITERIA FOR SCHIZOAFFECTIVE DISORDER

C9

A. An uninterrupted period of illness during which there is a major mood episode [a Manic Episode **(A40/A65)** or a Major Depressive Episode **(A12/A26)** with depressed mood (i.e., the episode is not limited to anhedonia)] concurrent with [symptoms that meet full] Criterion A of Schizophrenia **[C2]**. **Note:** The Major Depressive Episode must include Criterion A1: Depressed mood **[A1/A15]**.

NOTE: Code "YES" if Manic Episodes or Major Depressive Episodes With Depressed Mood are concurrent with Criterion A symptoms of Schizophrenia. Code "NO" if the only concurrent mood episodes are Major Depressive Episodes without depressed mood (i.e., with loss of interest only.)

YES

NO → Go to **C22** (Other Specified Psychotic Disorder), **page 42.** **C9**

C10

B. Delusions **[B1–B13]** or hallucinations **[B14–B19]** for 2 or more weeks in the absence of a major mood episode (depressive or manic) during the lifetime duration of the illness.

> *The following question may be asked for clarification:* **Thinking about your whole life from the time you first became ill until now, has there been any time when you had** (PSYCHOTIC SXS) **when you were not (depressed/high/irritable/OWN WORDS)?**

YES

NO → Go to **C22** (Other Specified Psychotic Disorder), **page 42.** **C10**

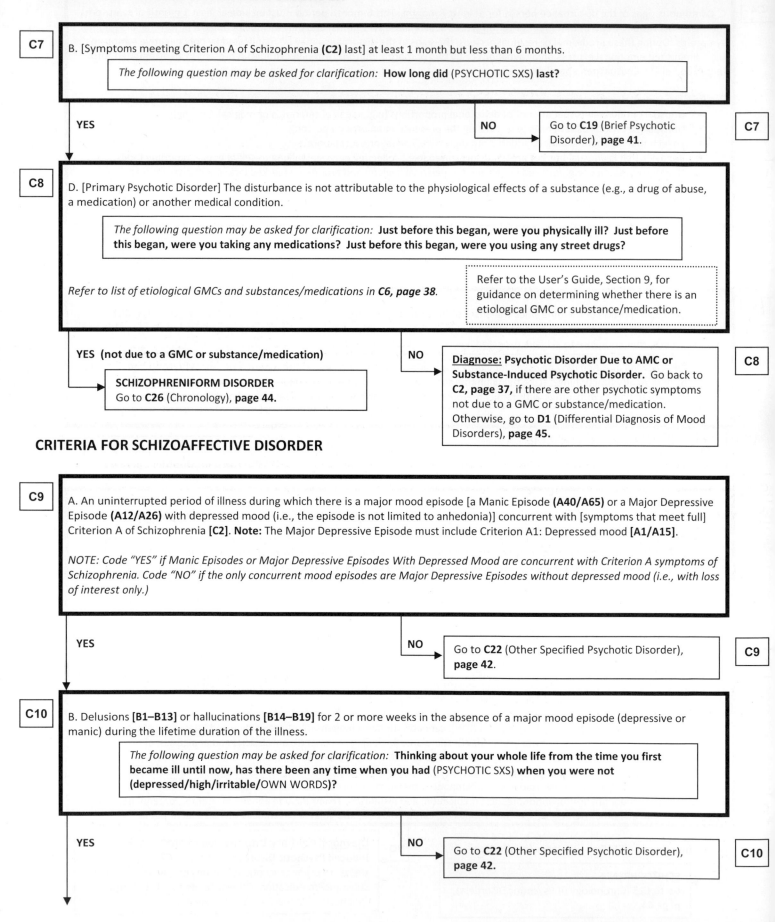

C11

C. Symptoms that meet criteria for a major mood episode are present for the majority [i.e., 50% or more] of the total duration of the active and residual portions of the illness.

> *The following question may be asked for clarification:* **How much of the time that you have had** (SXS FROM ACTIVE AND RESIDUAL PHASES) **would you say you have also been (depressed/high/irritable/**OWN WORDS**)?**

YES ↓   NO → | Go to **C22** Other Specified Psychotic Disorder), **page 42.**   **C11**

C12

D. [Primary Psychotic Disorder] The disturbance is not attributable to the physiological effects of a substance (e.g., a drug of abuse, a medication) or another medical condition.

> *The following question may be asked for clarification:* **Just before this began, were you physically ill? Just before this began, were you taking any medications? Just before this began, were you using any street drugs?**

Refer to list of etiological GMCs and substances/medications in C6, page 38.

> Refer to the User's Guide, Section 9, for guidance on determining whether there is an etiological GMC or substance/medication.

YES (not due to a GMC or substance/medication) ↓   NO →

SCHIZOAFFECTIVE DISORDER
Go to **C27** (Chronology of Psychotic Disorders), **page 44.**

| **Diagnose: Psychotic Disorder Due to AMC or Substance-Induced Psychotic Disorder.** Go back to **C2, page 37** if there are other psychotic symptoms not due to a GMC or substance/medication. Otherwise, go to **D1** (Differential Diagnosis of Mood Disorders), **page 45.**   **C12**

CRITERIA FOR DELUSIONAL DISORDER

C13

A. The presence of one (or more) delusions **[B1–B13]** with a duration of 1 month or longer.

NOTE: If delusions are restricted to beliefs about appearance or to beliefs about obsessions or compulsions, consider whether the delusions are better explained by a diagnosis of Body Dysmorphic Disorder or Obsessive-Compulsive Disorder, With Absent Insight/Delusional Beliefs. If so, skip to D1 (Differential Diagnosis of Mood Disorders), page 45.

YES ↓   NO → | Go to **C19** (Brief Psychotic Disorder), **page 41.**   **C13**

C14

B. Criterion A for Schizophrenia **[C2]** has never been met.
Note: Hallucinations, if present, are not prominent and are related to the delusional theme (e.g., the sensation of being infested with insects associated with delusions of infestation).

YES ↓   NO → | Go to **C22** (Other Specified Psychotic Disorder), **page 42.**   **C14**

C15

C. Apart from the impact of the delusion(s) or its ramifications, functioning is not markedly impaired, and behavior is not obviously bizarre or odd.

YES ↓   NO → | Go to **C22** (Other Specified Psychotic Disorder), **page 42.**   **C15**

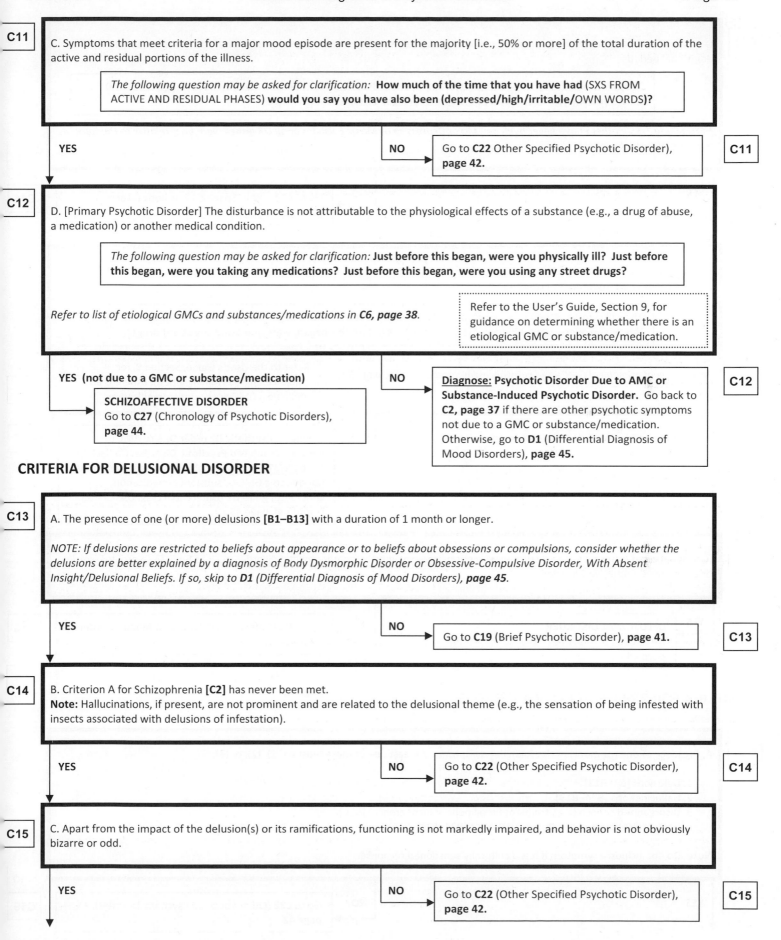

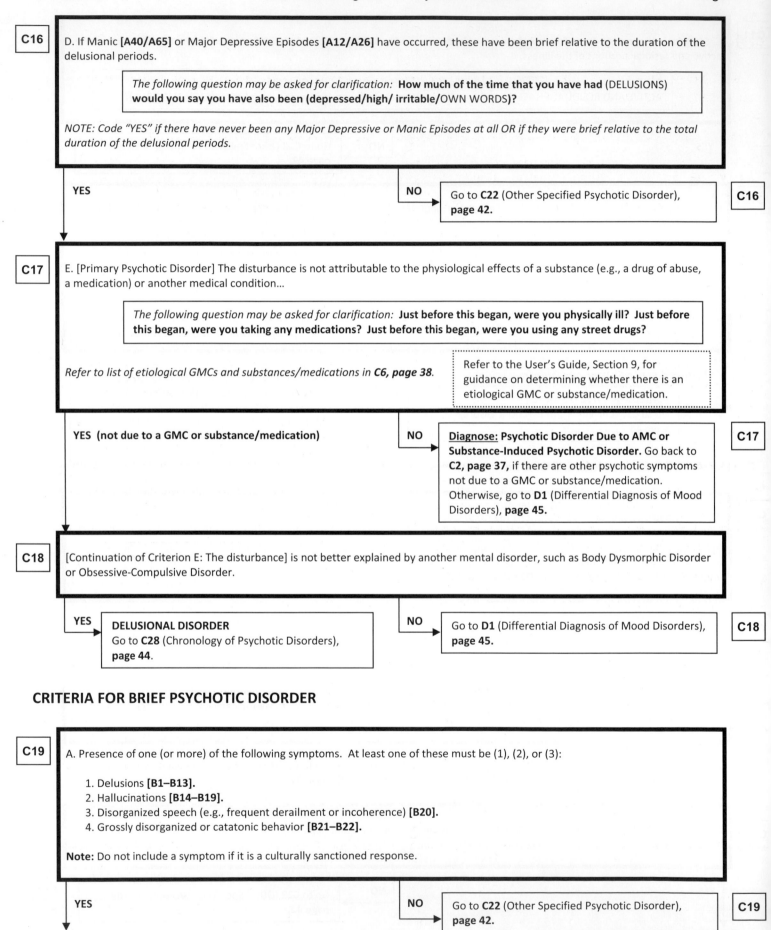

C16 D. If Manic **[A40/A65]** or Major Depressive Episodes **[A12/A26]** have occurred, these have been brief relative to the duration of the delusional periods.

> The following question may be asked for clarification: **How much of the time that you have had** (DELUSIONS) **would you say you have also been (depressed/high/ irritable/**OWN WORDS**)?**

NOTE: Code "YES" if there have never been any Major Depressive or Manic Episodes at all OR if they were brief relative to the total duration of the delusional periods.

YES

NO → Go to **C22** (Other Specified Psychotic Disorder), **page 42.** **C16**

C17 E. [Primary Psychotic Disorder] The disturbance is not attributable to the physiological effects of a substance (e.g., a drug of abuse, a medication) or another medical condition...

> The following question may be asked for clarification: **Just before this began, were you physically ill? Just before this began, were you taking any medications? Just before this began, were you using any street drugs?**

*Refer to list of etiological GMCs and substances/medications in **C6, page 38**.*

> Refer to the User's Guide, Section 9, for guidance on determining whether there is an etiological GMC or substance/medication.

YES (not due to a GMC or substance/medication)

NO → **Diagnose: Psychotic Disorder Due to AMC or Substance-Induced Psychotic Disorder.** Go back to **C2, page 37,** if there are other psychotic symptoms not due to a GMC or substance/medication. Otherwise, go to **D1** (Differential Diagnosis of Mood Disorders), **page 45.** **C17**

C18 [Continuation of Criterion E: The disturbance] is not better explained by another mental disorder, such as Body Dysmorphic Disorder or Obsessive-Compulsive Disorder.

YES → **DELUSIONAL DISORDER** Go to **C28** (Chronology of Psychotic Disorders), **page 44**.

NO → Go to **D1** (Differential Diagnosis of Mood Disorders), **page 45.** **C18**

CRITERIA FOR BRIEF PSYCHOTIC DISORDER

C19 A. Presence of one (or more) of the following symptoms. At least one of these must be (1), (2), or (3):

1. Delusions **[B1–B13].**
2. Hallucinations **[B14–B19].**
3. Disorganized speech (e.g., frequent derailment or incoherence) **[B20].**
4. Grossly disorganized or catatonic behavior **[B21–B22].**

Note: Do not include a symptom if it is a culturally sanctioned response.

YES

NO → Go to **C22** (Other Specified Psychotic Disorder), **page 42.** **C19**

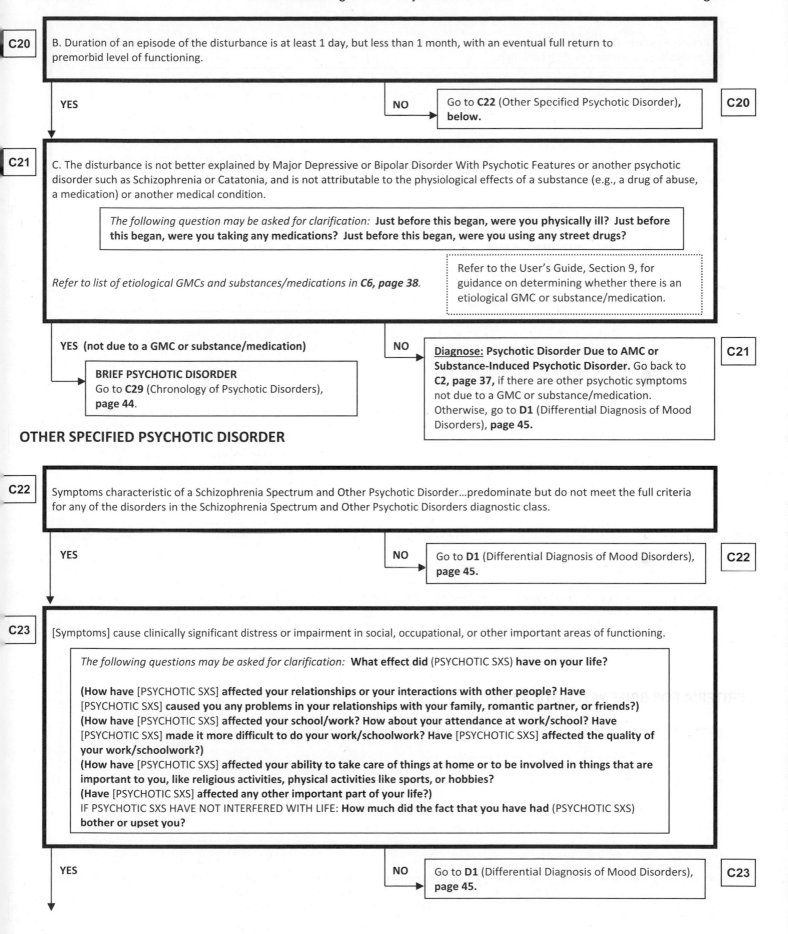

C20

B. Duration of an episode of the disturbance is at least 1 day, but less than 1 month, with an eventual full return to premorbid level of functioning.

YES   NO → Go to **C22** (Other Specified Psychotic Disorder), **below.**   **C20**

C21

C. The disturbance is not better explained by Major Depressive or Bipolar Disorder With Psychotic Features or another psychotic disorder such as Schizophrenia or Catatonia, and is not attributable to the physiological effects of a substance (e.g., a drug of abuse, a medication) or another medical condition.

> *The following question may be asked for clarification:* **Just before this began, were you physically ill? Just before this began, were you taking any medications? Just before this began, were you using any street drugs?**

*Refer to list of etiological GMCs and substances/medications in **C6, page 38**.*

> Refer to the User's Guide, Section 9, for guidance on determining whether there is an etiological GMC or substance/medication.

YES **(not due to a GMC or substance/medication)**   NO → **Diagnose: Psychotic Disorder Due to AMC or Substance-Induced Psychotic Disorder.** Go back to **C2, page 37,** if there are other psychotic symptoms not due to a GMC or substance/medication. Otherwise, go to **D1** (Differential Diagnosis of Mood Disorders), **page 45.**   **C21**

BRIEF PSYCHOTIC DISORDER
Go to **C29** (Chronology of Psychotic Disorders), **page 44**.

OTHER SPECIFIED PSYCHOTIC DISORDER

C22

Symptoms characteristic of a Schizophrenia Spectrum and Other Psychotic Disorder…predominate but do not meet the full criteria for any of the disorders in the Schizophrenia Spectrum and Other Psychotic Disorders diagnostic class.

YES   NO → Go to **D1** (Differential Diagnosis of Mood Disorders), **page 45.**   **C22**

C23

[Symptoms] cause clinically significant distress or impairment in social, occupational, or other important areas of functioning.

> *The following questions may be asked for clarification:* **What effect did** (PSYCHOTIC SXS) **have on your life?**
>
> **(How have** [PSYCHOTIC SXS] **affected your relationships or your interactions with other people? Have** [PSYCHOTIC SXS] **caused you any problems in your relationships with your family, romantic partner, or friends?)**
> **(How have** [PSYCHOTIC SXS] **affected your school/work? How about your attendance at work/school? Have** [PSYCHOTIC SXS] **made it more difficult to do your work/schoolwork? Have** [PSYCHOTIC SXS] **affected the quality of your work/schoolwork?)**
> **(How have** [PSYCHOTIC SXS] **affected your ability to take care of things at home or to be involved in things that are important to you, like religious activities, physical activities like sports, or hobbies?**
> **(Have** [PSYCHOTIC SXS] **affected any other important part of your life?)**
> IF PSYCHOTIC SXS HAVE NOT INTERFERED WITH LIFE: **How much did the fact that you have had** (PSYCHOTIC SXS) **bother or upset you?**

YES   NO → Go to **D1** (Differential Diagnosis of Mood Disorders), **page 45.**   **C23**

C24   [Primary Psychotic Disorder] The disturbance is not attributable to the physiological effects of a substance (e.g., a drug of abuse, a medication) or another medical condition.

> *The following question may be asked for clarification:* **Just before this began, were you physically ill? Just before this began, were you taking any medications? Just before this began, were you using any street drugs?**

Refer to list of etiological GMCs and substances/medications in **C6, page 38**.

> Refer to the User's Guide, Section 9, for guidance on determining whether there is an etiological GMC or substance/medication.

YES (not due to a GMC or substance/medication)

OTHER SPECIFIED PSYCHOTIC DISORDER
Go to **C30** (Chronology of Psychotic Disorders), **page 44.**

NO

<u>Diagnose:</u> **Psychotic Disorder Due to AMC or Substance-Induced Psychotic Disorder.** Go back to **C2, page 37,** if there are other psychotic symptoms not due to a GMC or substance/medication. Otherwise, go to **D1** (Differential Diagnosis of Mood Disorders), **page 45.**

C24

CHRONOLOGY OF PSYCHOTIC DISORDERS

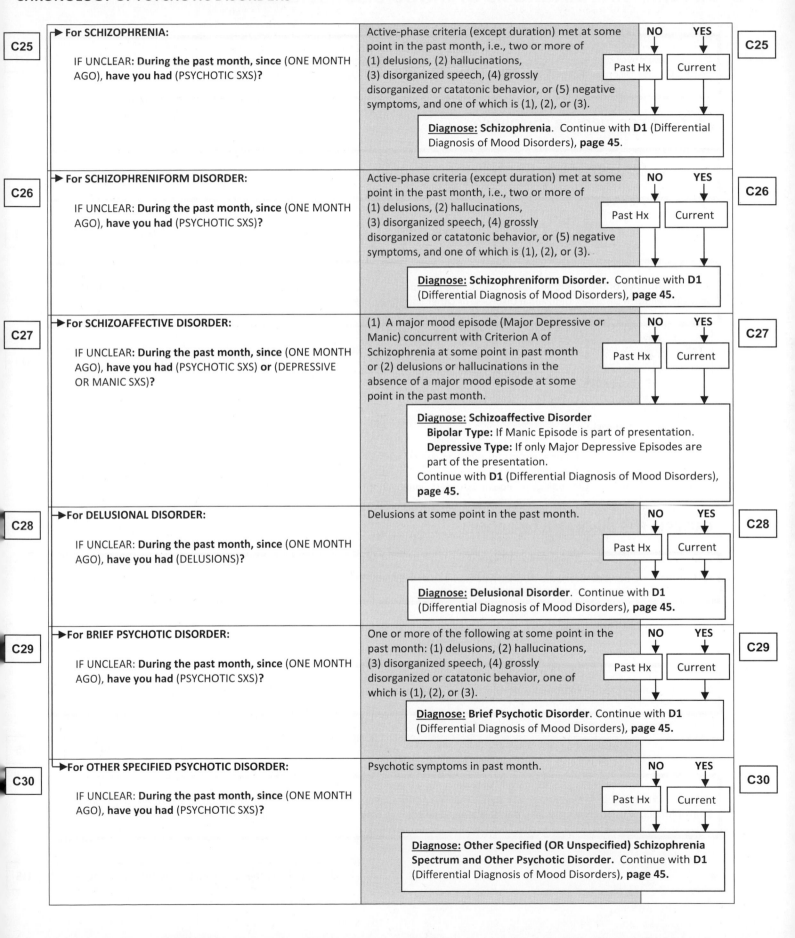

C25   For SCHIZOPHRENIA:

IF UNCLEAR: **During the past month, since** (ONE MONTH AGO), **have you had** (PSYCHOTIC SXS)?

Active-phase criteria (except duration) met at some point in the past month, i.e., two or more of (1) delusions, (2) hallucinations, (3) disorganized speech, (4) grossly disorganized or catatonic behavior, or (5) negative symptoms, and one of which is (1), (2), or (3).

NO → Past Hx   YES → Current   **C25**

Diagnose: Schizophrenia. Continue with **D1** (Differential Diagnosis of Mood Disorders), **page 45.**

C26   For SCHIZOPHRENIFORM DISORDER:

IF UNCLEAR: **During the past month, since** (ONE MONTH AGO), **have you had** (PSYCHOTIC SXS)?

Active-phase criteria (except duration) met at some point in the past month, i.e., two or more of (1) delusions, (2) hallucinations, (3) disorganized speech, (4) grossly disorganized or catatonic behavior, or (5) negative symptoms, and one of which is (1), (2), or (3).

NO → Past Hx   YES → Current   **C26**

Diagnose: Schizophreniform Disorder. Continue with **D1** (Differential Diagnosis of Mood Disorders), **page 45.**

C27   For SCHIZOAFFECTIVE DISORDER:

IF UNCLEAR: **During the past month, since** (ONE MONTH AGO), **have you had** (PSYCHOTIC SXS) **or** (DEPRESSIVE OR MANIC SXS)?

(1) A major mood episode (Major Depressive or Manic) concurrent with Criterion A of Schizophrenia at some point in past month or (2) delusions or hallucinations in the absence of a major mood episode at some point in the past month.

NO → Past Hx   YES → Current   **C27**

Diagnose: Schizoaffective Disorder
  Bipolar Type: If Manic Episode is part of presentation.
  Depressive Type: If only Major Depressive Episodes are part of the presentation.
Continue with **D1** (Differential Diagnosis of Mood Disorders), **page 45.**

C28   For DELUSIONAL DISORDER:

IF UNCLEAR: **During the past month, since** (ONE MONTH AGO), **have you had** (DELUSIONS)?

Delusions at some point in the past month.

NO → Past Hx   YES → Current   **C28**

Diagnose: Delusional Disorder. Continue with **D1** (Differential Diagnosis of Mood Disorders), **page 45.**

C29   For BRIEF PSYCHOTIC DISORDER:

IF UNCLEAR: **During the past month, since** (ONE MONTH AGO), **have you had** (PSYCHOTIC SXS)?

One or more of the following at some point in the past month: (1) delusions, (2) hallucinations, (3) disorganized speech, (4) grossly disorganized or catatonic behavior, one of which is (1), (2), or (3).

NO → Past Hx   YES → Current   **C29**

Diagnose: Brief Psychotic Disorder. Continue with **D1** (Differential Diagnosis of Mood Disorders), **page 45.**

C30   For OTHER SPECIFIED PSYCHOTIC DISORDER:

IF UNCLEAR: **During the past month, since** (ONE MONTH AGO), **have you had** (PSYCHOTIC SXS)?

Psychotic symptoms in past month.

NO → Past Hx   YES → Current   **C30**

Diagnose: Other Specified (OR Unspecified) Schizophrenia Spectrum and Other Psychotic Disorder. Continue with **D1** (Differential Diagnosis of Mood Disorders), **page 45.**

D. DIFFERENTIAL DIAGNOSIS OF MOOD DISORDERS

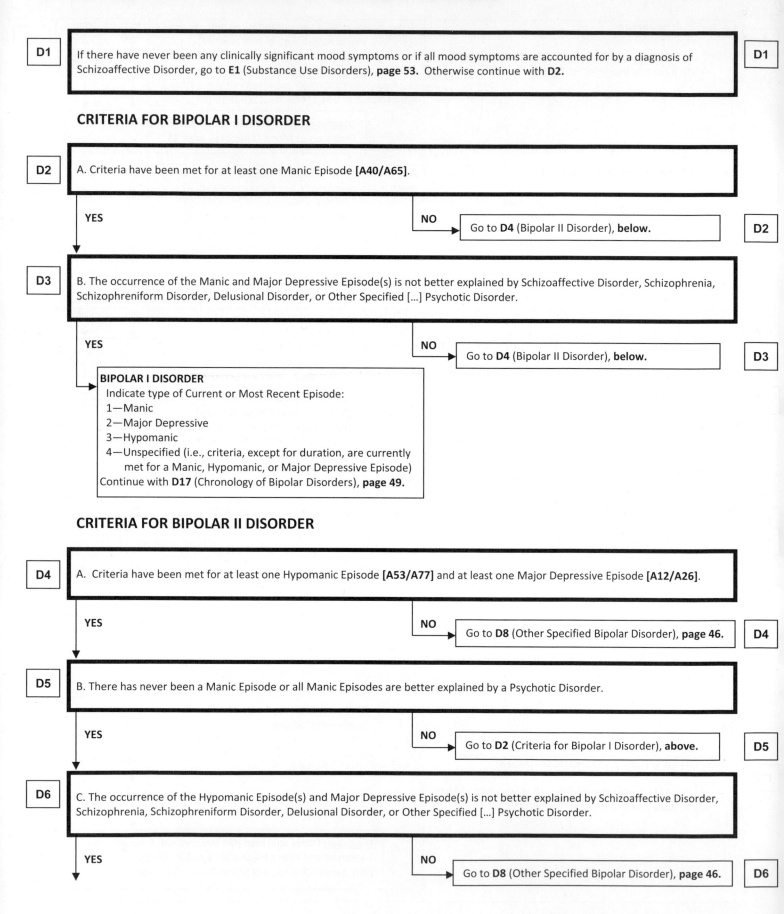

D1   If there have never been any clinically significant mood symptoms or if all mood symptoms are accounted for by a diagnosis of Schizoaffective Disorder, go to **E1** (Substance Use Disorders), **page 53.** Otherwise continue with **D2.**   **D1**

CRITERIA FOR BIPOLAR I DISORDER

D2   A. Criteria have been met for at least one Manic Episode **[A40/A65].**

YES   NO → Go to **D4** (Bipolar II Disorder), **below.**   **D2**

D3   B. The occurrence of the Manic and Major Depressive Episode(s) is not better explained by Schizoaffective Disorder, Schizophrenia, Schizophreniform Disorder, Delusional Disorder, or Other Specified [...] Psychotic Disorder.

YES   NO → Go to **D4** (Bipolar II Disorder), **below.**   **D3**

BIPOLAR I DISORDER
Indicate type of Current or Most Recent Episode:
1—Manic
2—Major Depressive
3—Hypomanic
4—Unspecified (i.e., criteria, except for duration, are currently met for a Manic, Hypomanic, or Major Depressive Episode)
Continue with **D17** (Chronology of Bipolar Disorders), **page 49.**

CRITERIA FOR BIPOLAR II DISORDER

D4   A. Criteria have been met for at least one Hypomanic Episode **[A53/A77]** and at least one Major Depressive Episode **[A12/A26].**

YES   NO → Go to **D8** (Other Specified Bipolar Disorder), **page 46.**   **D4**

D5   B. There has never been a Manic Episode or all Manic Episodes are better explained by a Psychotic Disorder.

YES   NO → Go to **D2** (Criteria for Bipolar I Disorder), **above.**   **D5**

D6   C. The occurrence of the Hypomanic Episode(s) and Major Depressive Episode(s) is not better explained by Schizoaffective Disorder, Schizophrenia, Schizophreniform Disorder, Delusional Disorder, or Other Specified [...] Psychotic Disorder.

YES   NO → Go to **D8** (Other Specified Bipolar Disorder), **page 46.**   **D6**

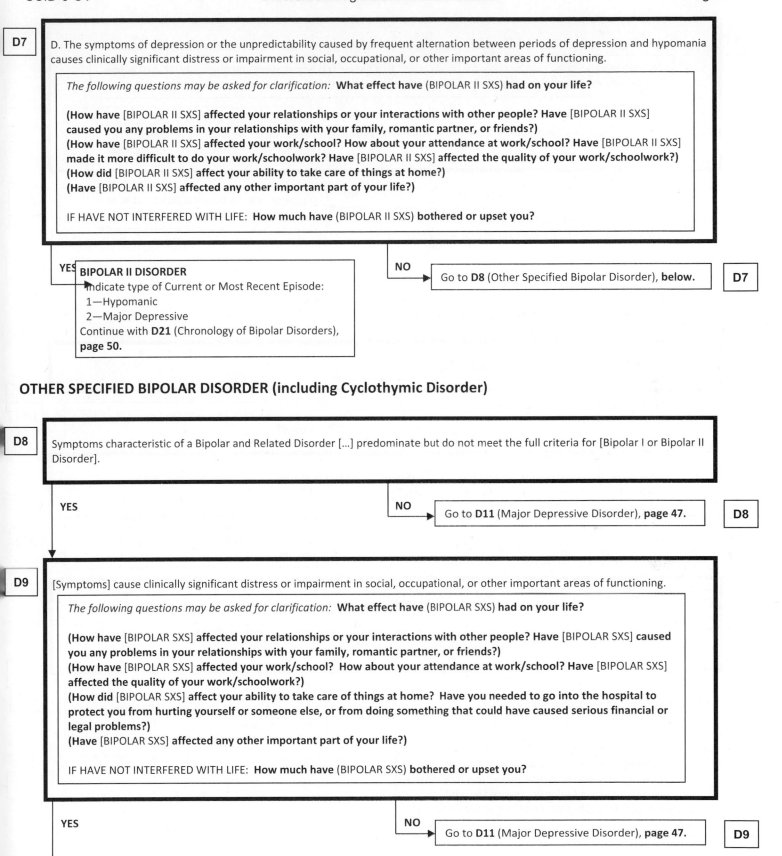

D7

D. The symptoms of depression or the unpredictability caused by frequent alternation between periods of depression and hypomania causes clinically significant distress or impairment in social, occupational, or other important areas of functioning.

> *The following questions may be asked for clarification:* **What effect have (BIPOLAR II SXS) had on your life?**
>
> **(How have** [BIPOLAR II SXS] **affected your relationships or your interactions with other people? Have** [BIPOLAR II SXS] **caused you any problems in your relationships with your family, romantic partner, or friends?)**
> **(How have** [BIPOLAR II SXS] **affected your work/school? How about your attendance at work/school? Have** [BIPOLAR II SXS] **made it more difficult to do your work/schoolwork? Have** [BIPOLAR II SXS] **affected the quality of your work/schoolwork?)**
> **(How did** [BIPOLAR II SXS] **affect your ability to take care of things at home?)**
> **(Have** [BIPOLAR II SXS] **affected any other important part of your life?)**
>
> IF HAVE NOT INTERFERED WITH LIFE: **How much have (BIPOLAR II SXS) bothered or upset you?**

YES

BIPOLAR II DISORDER
Indicate type of Current or Most Recent Episode:
1—Hypomanic
2—Major Depressive
Continue with **D21** (Chronology of Bipolar Disorders), **page 50.**

NO → Go to **D8** (Other Specified Bipolar Disorder), **below.**   **D7**

OTHER SPECIFIED BIPOLAR DISORDER (including Cyclothymic Disorder)

D8

Symptoms characteristic of a Bipolar and Related Disorder [...] predominate but do not meet the full criteria for [Bipolar I or Bipolar II Disorder].

YES

NO → Go to **D11** (Major Depressive Disorder), **page 47.**   **D8**

D9

[Symptoms] cause clinically significant distress or impairment in social, occupational, or other important areas of functioning.

> *The following questions may be asked for clarification:* **What effect have (BIPOLAR SXS) had on your life?**
>
> **(How have** [BIPOLAR SXS] **affected your relationships or your interactions with other people? Have** [BIPOLAR SXS] **caused you any problems in your relationships with your family, romantic partner, or friends?)**
> **(How have** [BIPOLAR SXS] **affected your work/school? How about your attendance at work/school? Have** [BIPOLAR SXS] **affected the quality of your work/schoolwork?)**
> **(How did** [BIPOLAR SXS] **affect your ability to take care of things at home? Have you needed to go into the hospital to protect you from hurting yourself or someone else, or from doing something that could have caused serious financial or legal problems?)**
> **(Have** [BIPOLAR SXS] **affected any other important part of your life?)**
>
> IF HAVE NOT INTERFERED WITH LIFE: **How much have (BIPOLAR SXS) bothered or upset you?**

YES

NO → Go to **D11** (Major Depressive Disorder), **page 47.**   **D9**

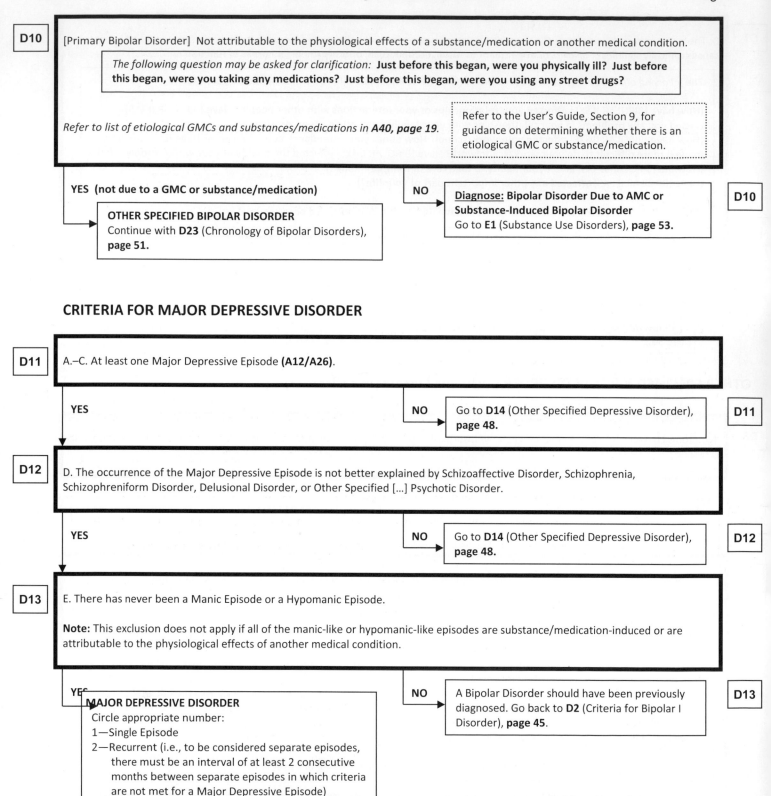

D10 [Primary Bipolar Disorder] Not attributable to the physiological effects of a substance/medication or another medical condition.

> *The following question may be asked for clarification:* **Just before this began, were you physically ill? Just before this began, were you taking any medications? Just before this began, were you using any street drugs?**

*Refer to list of etiological GMCs and substances/medications in **A40, page 19**.*

> Refer to the User's Guide, Section 9, for guidance on determining whether there is an etiological GMC or substance/medication.

YES (not due to a GMC or substance/medication)

> **OTHER SPECIFIED BIPOLAR DISORDER**
> Continue with **D23** (Chronology of Bipolar Disorders), **page 51.**

NO

> **Diagnose: Bipolar Disorder Due to AMC or Substance-Induced Bipolar Disorder**
> Go to **E1** (Substance Use Disorders), **page 53.**   **D10**

CRITERIA FOR MAJOR DEPRESSIVE DISORDER

D11 A.–C. At least one Major Depressive Episode **(A12/A26)**.

YES

NO   Go to **D14** (Other Specified Depressive Disorder), **page 48.**   **D11**

D12 D. The occurrence of the Major Depressive Episode is not better explained by Schizoaffective Disorder, Schizophrenia, Schizophreniform Disorder, Delusional Disorder, or Other Specified [...] Psychotic Disorder.

YES

NO   Go to **D14** (Other Specified Depressive Disorder), **page 48.**   **D12**

D13 E. There has never been a Manic Episode or a Hypomanic Episode.

Note: This exclusion does not apply if all of the manic-like or hypomanic-like episodes are substance/medication-induced or are attributable to the physiological effects of another medical condition.

YES

> **MAJOR DEPRESSIVE DISORDER**
> Circle appropriate number:
> 1—Single Episode
> 2—Recurrent (i.e., to be considered separate episodes, there must be an interval of at least 2 consecutive months between separate episodes in which criteria are not met for a Major Depressive Episode)
> Continue with **D24** (Chronology of Depressive Disorders), **page 52.**

NO   A Bipolar Disorder should have been previously diagnosed. Go back to **D2** (Criteria for Bipolar I Disorder), **page 45.**   **D13**

OTHER SPECIFIED DEPRESSIVE DISORDER

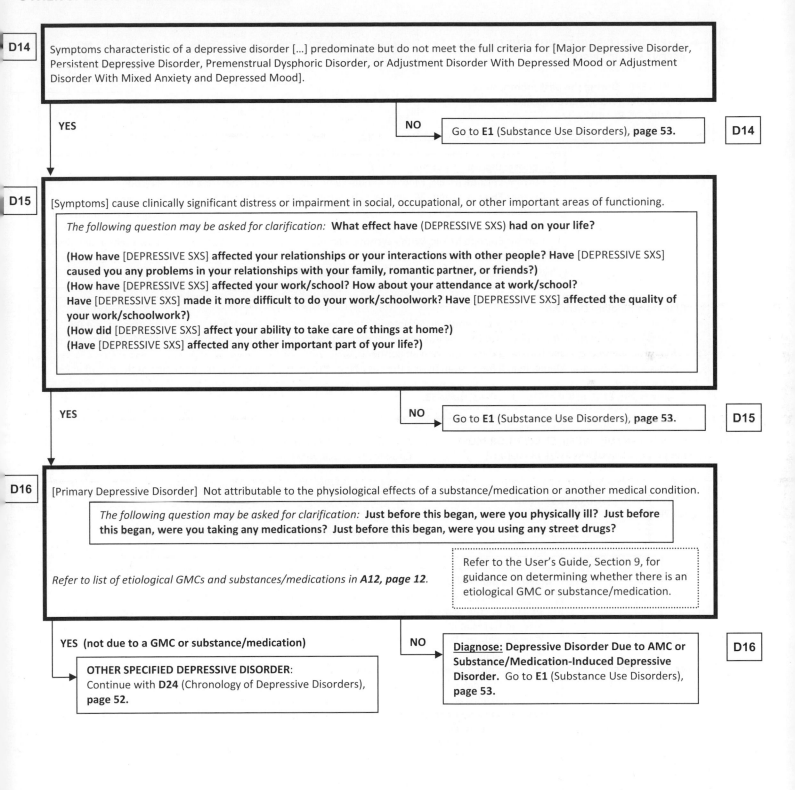

D14 Symptoms characteristic of a depressive disorder [...] predominate but do not meet the full criteria for [Major Depressive Disorder, Persistent Depressive Disorder, Premenstrual Dysphoric Disorder, or Adjustment Disorder With Depressed Mood or Adjustment Disorder With Mixed Anxiety and Depressed Mood].

YES

NO → Go to **E1** (Substance Use Disorders), **page 53.**   **D14**

D15 [Symptoms] cause clinically significant distress or impairment in social, occupational, or other important areas of functioning.

The following question may be asked for clarification: **What effect have** (DEPRESSIVE SXS) **had on your life?**

(How have [DEPRESSIVE SXS] **affected your relationships or your interactions with other people? Have** [DEPRESSIVE SXS] **caused you any problems in your relationships with your family, romantic partner, or friends?)**
(How have [DEPRESSIVE SXS] **affected your work/school? How about your attendance at work/school?**
Have [DEPRESSIVE SXS] **made it more difficult to do your work/schoolwork? Have** [DEPRESSIVE SXS] **affected the quality of your work/schoolwork?)**
(How did [DEPRESSIVE SXS] **affect your ability to take care of things at home?)**
(Have [DEPRESSIVE SXS] **affected any other important part of your life?)**

YES

NO → Go to **E1** (Substance Use Disorders), **page 53.**   **D15**

D16 [Primary Depressive Disorder] Not attributable to the physiological effects of a substance/medication or another medical condition.

The following question may be asked for clarification: **Just before this began, were you physically ill? Just before this began, were you taking any medications? Just before this began, were you using any street drugs?**

*Refer to list of etiological GMCs and substances/medications in **A12, page 12**.*

Refer to the User's Guide, Section 9, for guidance on determining whether there is an etiological GMC or substance/medication.

YES **(not due to a GMC or substance/medication)**

OTHER SPECIFIED DEPRESSIVE DISORDER:
Continue with **D24** (Chronology of Depressive Disorders), **page 52.**

NO → **Diagnose: Depressive Disorder Due to AMC or Substance/Medication-Induced Depressive Disorder.** Go to **E1** (Substance Use Disorders), **page 53.**   **D16**

CHRONOLOGY OF BIPOLAR DISORDERS

D17   → For <u>BIPOLAR I DISORDER,</u> **CURRENT OR MOST RECENT MANIC EPISODE:**

IF UNCLEAR: **During the past month, since (ONE MONTH AGO), have you had (MANIC SXS RATED "+")?**

Has met symptomatic criteria for a Manic Episode in the past month.

NO   **YES**   **D**

| Past Hx | Current |

Diagnose: Bipolar I Disorder
 Current Episode Manic, Mild: Minimum symptom criteria are met for a Manic Episode.
 Current Episode Manic, Moderate: Extreme increase in activity or impairment in judgment.
 Current Episode Manic, Severe: Almost continual supervision is required in order to prevent physical harm to self or others.
 Current Episode Manic, With Psychotic Features: Delusions or hallucinations are present at any time in the episode.
Continue with **E1** (Substance Use Disorders), **page 53**.

Diagnose: Bipolar I Disorder
 Most Recent Episode Manic, In Partial Remission: Symptoms of the immediate previous Manic Episode are present, but full criteria are not met, or there is a period lasting less than 2 months without any significant symptoms of a Manic, Hypomanic, or Major Depressive Episode following the end of such an episode.
 Most Recent Episode Manic, In Full Remission: During the past 2 months, no significant signs or symptoms of the disturbance were present.
Continue with **E1** (Substance Use Disorders), **page 53**.

D18   → For <u>BIPOLAR I DISORDER,</u> **CURRENT OR MOST RECENT MAJOR DEPRESSIVE EPISODE:**

IF UNCLEAR: **During the past month, since (ONE MONTH AGO), have you had (DEPRESSIVE SXS RATED "+")?**

Has met symptomatic criteria for a Major Depressive Episode in the past month.

*NOTE: If full criteria have been simultaneously met for both a current Manic Episode and a current Major Depressive Episode, the individual is considered to have a current Manic Episode (rated above in **D17**) and not a current Major Depressive Episode.*

NO   **YES**   **D**

| Past Hx | Current |

Diagnose: Bipolar I Disorder
 Current Episode Depressed, Mild: Few, if any, symptoms in excess of those required to meet the diagnostic criteria are present, the intensity of the symptoms is distressing but manageable, and the symptoms result in minor impairment in social or occupational functioning.
 Current Episode Depressed, Moderate: The number of symptoms, intensity of symptoms, and/or functional impairment is between those specified for "mild" and "severe."
 Current Episode Depressed, Severe: The number of symptoms is substantially in excess of those required to make the diagnosis, the intensity of the symptoms is seriously distressing and unmanageable, and the symptoms markedly interfere with social and occupational functioning.
 Current Episode Depressed, With Psychotic Features: Delusions or hallucinations are present at any time in the episode.
Continue with **E1** (Substance Use Disorders), **page 53**.

Diagnose: Bipolar I Disorder
 Most Recent Episode Depressed, In Partial Remission: Symptoms of the immediate previous Major Depressive Episode are present, but full criteria are not met, or there is a period lasting less than 2 months without any significant symptoms of a Manic, Hypomanic, or Major Depressive Episode following the end of such an episode.
 Most Recent Episode Depressed, In Full Remission: During the past 2 months, no significant signs or symptoms of the disturbance were present.
Continue with **E1** (Substance Use Disorders), **page 53**.

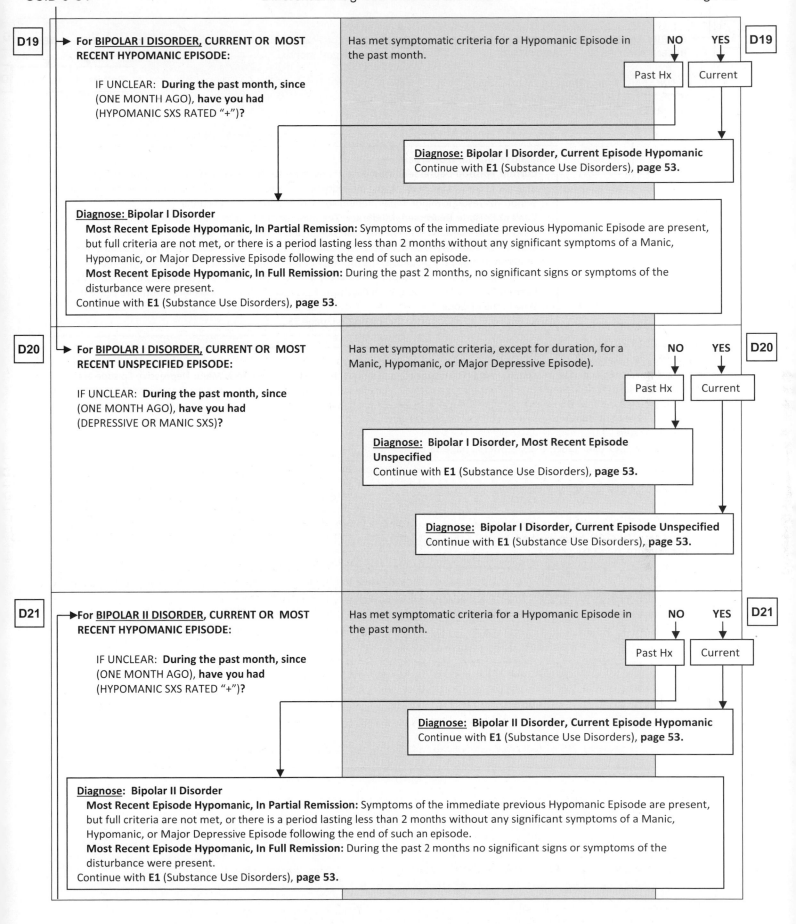

D19 → For <u>BIPOLAR I DISORDER,</u> CURRENT OR MOST RECENT HYPOMANIC EPISODE:

IF UNCLEAR: **During the past month, since** (ONE MONTH AGO), **have you had** (HYPOMANIC SXS RATED "+")**?**

Has met symptomatic criteria for a Hypomanic Episode in the past month.

NO   YES   **D19**

Past Hx   Current

Diagnose: Bipolar I Disorder, Current Episode Hypomanic
Continue with **E1** (Substance Use Disorders), **page 53.**

Diagnose: Bipolar I Disorder
Most Recent Episode Hypomanic, In Partial Remission: Symptoms of the immediate previous Hypomanic Episode are present, but full criteria are not met, or there is a period lasting less than 2 months without any significant symptoms of a Manic, Hypomanic, or Major Depressive Episode following the end of such an episode.
Most Recent Episode Hypomanic, In Full Remission: During the past 2 months, no significant signs or symptoms of the disturbance were present.
Continue with **E1** (Substance Use Disorders), **page 53.**

D20 → For <u>BIPOLAR I DISORDER,</u> CURRENT OR MOST RECENT UNSPECIFIED EPISODE:

IF UNCLEAR: **During the past month, since** (ONE MONTH AGO), **have you had** (DEPRESSIVE OR MANIC SXS)**?**

Has met symptomatic criteria, except for duration, for a Manic, Hypomanic, or Major Depressive Episode).

NO   YES   **D20**

Past Hx   Current

Diagnose: Bipolar I Disorder, Most Recent Episode Unspecified
Continue with **E1** (Substance Use Disorders), **page 53.**

Diagnose: Bipolar I Disorder, Current Episode Unspecified
Continue with **E1** (Substance Use Disorders), **page 53.**

D21 → For <u>BIPOLAR II DISORDER,</u> CURRENT OR MOST RECENT HYPOMANIC EPISODE:

IF UNCLEAR: **During the past month, since** (ONE MONTH AGO), **have you had** (HYPOMANIC SXS RATED "+")**?**

Has met symptomatic criteria for a Hypomanic Episode in the past month.

NO   YES   **D21**

Past Hx   Current

Diagnose: Bipolar II Disorder, Current Episode Hypomanic
Continue with **E1** (Substance Use Disorders), **page 53.**

Diagnose: Bipolar II Disorder
Most Recent Episode Hypomanic, In Partial Remission: Symptoms of the immediate previous Hypomanic Episode are present, but full criteria are not met, or there is a period lasting less than 2 months without any significant symptoms of a Manic, Hypomanic, or Major Depressive Episode following the end of such an episode.
Most Recent Episode Hypomanic, In Full Remission: During the past 2 months no significant signs or symptoms of the disturbance were present.
Continue with **E1** (Substance Use Disorders), **page 53.**

D22   → For <u>BIPOLAR II DISORDER,</u> CURRENT OR MOST RECENT MAJOR DEPRESSIVE EPISODE:

IF UNCLEAR: **During the past month, since (ONE MONTH AGO), have you had (DEPRESSIVE SXS RATED "+")?**

Has met symptomatic criteria for a Major Depressive Episode in the past month.

NO   **YES**

Past Hx   Current

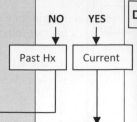

Diagnose: Bipolar II Disorder

Current Episode Depressed, Mild: Few, if any, symptoms in excess of those required to meet the diagnostic criteria are present, the intensity of the symptoms is distressing but manageable, and the symptoms result in minor impairment in social or occupational functioning.

Current Episode Depressed, Moderate: The number of symptoms, intensity of symptoms, and/or functional impairment is between those specified for "mild" and "severe."

Current Episode Depressed, Severe: The number of symptoms is substantially in excess of those required to make the diagnosis, the intensity of the symptoms is seriously distressing and unmanageable, and the symptoms markedly interfere with social and occupational functioning.

Current Episode Depressed, With Psychotic Features: Delusions or hallucinations are present at any time in the episode.

Continue with **E1** (Substance Use Disorders), **page 53.**

Diagnose: Bipolar II Disorder

Most Recent Episode Depressed, In Partial Remission: Symptoms of the immediate previous Major Depressive Episode are present, but full criteria are not met, or there is a period lasting less than 2 months without any significant symptoms of a Manic, Hypomanic, or Major Depressive Episode following the end of such an episode.

Most Recent Episode Depressed, In Full Remission: During the past 2 months no significant signs or symptoms of the disturbance were present.

Continue with **E1** (Substance Use Disorders), **page 53.**

D23   → For OTHER SPECIFIED BIPOLAR DISORDER:

IF UNCLEAR: **During the past month, since (ONE MONTH AGO), have you had (DEPRESSIVE OR MANIC SXS)?**

Symptoms characteristic of a Bipolar and Related Disorder causing clinically significant distress or impairment are present in the past month.

NO   **YES**

Past Hx   Current

Diagnose: Other Specified (OR Unspecified) Bipolar and Related Disorder

Continue with **E1** (Substance Use Disorders), **page 53.**

CHRONOLOGY OF DEPRESSIVE DISORDERS

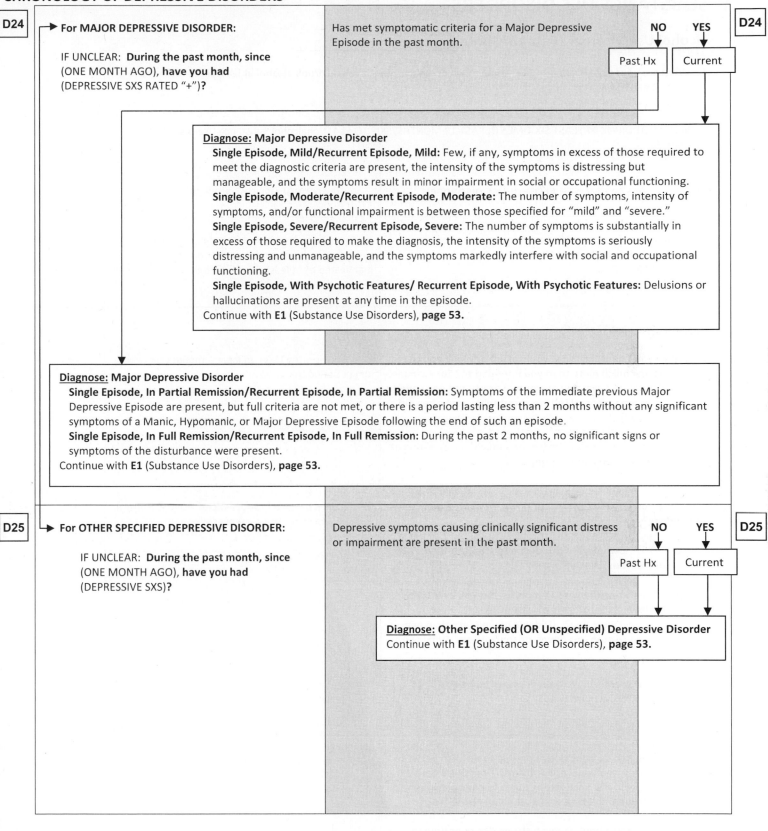

D24

→ **For MAJOR DEPRESSIVE DISORDER:**

IF UNCLEAR: **During the past month, since (ONE MONTH AGO), have you had (DEPRESSIVE SXS RATED "+")?**

Has met symptomatic criteria for a Major Depressive Episode in the past month.

NO   YES

Past Hx   Current

D24

Diagnose: Major Depressive Disorder
Single Episode, Mild/Recurrent Episode, Mild: Few, if any, symptoms in excess of those required to meet the diagnostic criteria are present, the intensity of the symptoms is distressing but manageable, and the symptoms result in minor impairment in social or occupational functioning.
Single Episode, Moderate/Recurrent Episode, Moderate: The number of symptoms, intensity of symptoms, and/or functional impairment is between those specified for "mild" and "severe."
Single Episode, Severe/Recurrent Episode, Severe: The number of symptoms is substantially in excess of those required to make the diagnosis, the intensity of the symptoms is seriously distressing and unmanageable, and the symptoms markedly interfere with social and occupational functioning.
Single Episode, With Psychotic Features/ Recurrent Episode, With Psychotic Features: Delusions or hallucinations are present at any time in the episode.
Continue with **E1** (Substance Use Disorders), **page 53.**

Diagnose: Major Depressive Disorder
Single Episode, In Partial Remission/Recurrent Episode, In Partial Remission: Symptoms of the immediate previous Major Depressive Episode are present, but full criteria are not met, or there is a period lasting less than 2 months without any significant symptoms of a Manic, Hypomanic, or Major Depressive Episode following the end of such an episode.
Single Episode, In Full Remission/Recurrent Episode, In Full Remission: During the past 2 months, no significant signs or symptoms of the disturbance were present.
Continue with **E1** (Substance Use Disorders), **page 53.**

D25

→ **For OTHER SPECIFIED DEPRESSIVE DISORDER:**

IF UNCLEAR: **During the past month, since (ONE MONTH AGO), have you had (DEPRESSIVE SXS)?**

Depressive symptoms causing clinically significant distress or impairment are present in the past month.

NO   YES

Past Hx   Current

D25

Diagnose: Other Specified (OR Unspecified) Depressive Disorder
Continue with **E1** (Substance Use Disorders), **page 53.**

E. SUBSTANCE USE DISORDERS

Alcohol Use Disorder (Past 12 Months)

<table>
<tr>
<td>E1</td>
<td colspan="2">What are your drinking habits like? (How much do you drink? Have you drunk alcohol at least six times in the past 12 months, that is, since (ONE YEAR AGO)?

IF DID NOT DRINK AT LEAST SIX TIMES IN PAST 12 MONTHS, SKIP TO E14 (Nonalcohol Substance Use Disorder), page 56.</td>
<td>E1</td>
</tr>
<tr>
<td></td>
<td align="center">PAST-12-MONTH ALCOHOL USE DISORDER</td>
<td>ALCOHOL USE DISORDER CRITERIA</td>
<td></td>
</tr>
<tr>
<td></td>
<td>I'd now like to ask you some more questions about your drinking habits in the past 12 months, since (ONE YEAR AGO)….</td>
<td>A. A problematic pattern of alcohol use leading to clinically significant impairment or distress, as manifested by at least two of the following occurring within a 12-month period:</td>
<td></td>
</tr>
<tr>
<td>E2</td>
<td>During the past 12 months…

…have you found that once you started drinking you ended up drinking much more than you <u>intended</u> to? For example, you planned to have only one or two drinks but you ended up having many more. (Tell me about that. How often did this happen?)

IF NO: What about drinking for a much longer period of time than you were <u>intending</u> to?</td>
<td>1. Alcohol is often taken in larger amounts OR over a longer period than was intended.</td>
<td>—   +

E2</td>
</tr>
<tr>
<td>E3</td>
<td>…have you wanted to stop, cut down, or control your drinking?

IF YES: How long did this desire to stop, cut down, or control your drinking last?

IF NO: During the past 12 months, did you ever try to cut down, stop, or control your drinking? How successful were you? (Did you make more than one attempt to stop, cut down, or control your drinking?)</td>
<td>2. There is a persistent desire OR unsuccessful efforts to cut down or control alcohol use.</td>
<td>—   +

E3</td>
</tr>
<tr>
<td>E4</td>
<td>…have you spent a lot of time drinking, being drunk, or hung over? (How much time?)</td>
<td>3. A great deal of time is spent in activities necessary to obtain alcohol, use alcohol, or recover from its effects.</td>
<td>—   +

E4</td>
</tr>
<tr>
<td>E5</td>
<td>…have you had a strong desire or urge to drink In between those times when you were drinking? (Has there been a time when you had such strong urges to have a drink that you had trouble thinking about anything else?)

IF NO: How about having a strong desire or urge to drink when you were around bars or around people with whom you go drinking?</td>
<td>4. Craving, or a strong desire or urge to use alcohol.</td>
<td>—   +

E5</td>
</tr>
</table>

E6	**During the past 12 months, since** (ONE YEAR AGO)… …**have you missed work or school or often arrived late because you were intoxicated, high, or very hung over?** IF NO: **How about doing a bad job at work or school, or failing courses or getting kicked out of school because of your drinking?** IF NO: **How about getting into trouble at work or school because of your use of alcohol?** IF NO: **How about not taking care of things at home because of your drinking, like making sure there are food and clean clothes for your family and making sure your children go to school and get medical care? How about not paying your bills?** IF YES TO ANY: **How often?**	5. Recurrent alcohol use resulting in a failure to fulfill major role obligations at work, school, or home [e.g., repeated absences or poor work performance related to alcohol use; alcohol-related absences, suspensions, or expulsions from school; neglect of children or household].	—	+	**E6**
E7	…**has your drinking caused problems with other people, such as family members, friends, or people at work? (Have you found yourself regularly getting into arguments about what happens when you drink too much? Have you gotten into physical fights when you were drunk?)** IF YES: **Did you keep on drinking anyway? (Over what period of time?)**	6. Continued alcohol use despite having persistent or recurrent social or interpersonal problems caused or exacerbated by the effects of alcohol [e.g., arguments with spouse about consequences of intoxication, physical fights].	—	+	**E7**
E8	…**have you had to give up or reduce the time you spent at work or school, with family or friends, or on things you like to do (like sports, cooking, other hobbies) because you were drinking or hungover?**	7. Important social, occupational, or recreational activities are given up or reduced because of alcohol use.	—	+	**E8**
E9	…**have you ever had a few drinks right before doing something that requires coordination and concentration like driving, boating, climbing on a ladder, or operating heavy machinery?** IF YES: **Would you say that the amount you had to drink affected your coordination or concentration so that it was more likely that you or someone else could have been hurt?** IF YES AND UNKNOWN: **How many times? (When?)**	8. Recurrent alcohol use in situations in which it is physically hazardous [e.g., driving an automobile or operating a machine when impaired by alcohol use].	—	+	**E9**
E10	…**has your drinking caused you any problems like making you very depressed or anxious? How about putting you in a "mental fog," making it difficult for you to sleep, or making it so you couldn't recall what happened while you were drinking?** **Has your drinking caused significant physical problems or made a physical problem worse, like stomach ulcers, liver disease, or pancreatitis?** IF YES TO EITHER OF ABOVE: **Did you keep on drinking anyway?**	9. Alcohol use is continued despite knowledge of having a persistent or recurrent physical or psychological problem that is likely to have been caused or exacerbated by alcohol [e.g., continued drinking despite recognition that an ulcer was made worse by alcohol consumption].	—	+	**E10**

E11	During the past 12 months, since (ONE YEAR AGO)…
	
	…have you ever found that you needed to drink much more in order to get the feeling you wanted than you did when you first started drinking?
	
	➤ IF YES: How much more?
	
	➤ IF NO: What about finding that when you drank the same amount, it had much less effect than before? (How much less?)
		10. Tolerance, as defined by either of the following:
		
		    a. A need for markedly increased amounts of alcohol to achieve intoxication or desired effect.
		
		    b. A markedly diminished effect with continued use of the same amount of alcohol.
			— +	E1

E12	…have you ever had any withdrawal symptoms, in other words felt sick when you cut down or stopped drinking?
	
	➤ IF YES: What symptoms did you have? (Sweating or a racing heart? Your hand[s] shaking? Trouble sleeping? Feeling nauseated or vomiting? Feeling agitated? Feeling anxious? How about having a seizure or seeing, feeling, or hearing things that weren't really there?)
	
	➤ IF NO: Have you ever started the day with a drink, or did you often drink or take some other drug or medication to keep yourself from getting the shakes or becoming sick?
		11. Withdrawal, as manifested by either of the following:
		
		    a. [At least TWO] of the following, developing within several hours to a few days after the cessation of (or reduction in) alcohol use that has been heavy and prolonged:
		
		    1. Autonomic hyperactivity (e.g., sweating or pulse rate greater than 100 bpm)
		    2. Increased hand tremor
		    3. Insomnia
		    4. Nausea or vomiting
		    5. Transient visual, tactile, or auditory hallucinations or illusions
		    6. Psychomotor agitation
		    7. Anxiety
		    8. Generalized tonic-clonic seizures
		
		    b. Alcohol (or a closely related substance, such as a benzodiazepine) is taken to relieve or avoid withdrawal symptoms.
			— +	E1

E13	IF UNCLEAR: When did (ABOVE CRITERION A SXS [E2–E12] RATED "+") occur? (Did they all happen within the past 12 months?)	AT LEAST TWO OF THE ABOVE ALCOHOL USE CRITERION A SXS (E2–E12) ARE RATED "+" AND SXS OCCURRED WITHIN THE PAST 12 MONTHS.	NO YES	E1

Go to E14 (Nonalcohol Substance Use Disorder), page 56.

Diagnose: Alcohol Use Disorder
  Mild: If 2–3 symptoms.
  Moderate: If 4–5 symptoms.
  Severe: If 6 or more symptoms.
Continue with E14 (Nonalcohol Substance Use Disorder), page 56.

Nonalcohol Substance Use Disorder (Past 12 Months)

		DRUG CLASS USED IN PAST 12 MONTHS		
E14	Now I'd like to ask you about your use of drugs or medicines over the past 12 months, since (ONE YEAR AGO).			**E14**
	Drug Classes to Ask About			
E15	**Sedatives, Hypnotics, or Anxiolytics:** In the past 12 months, have you taken any pills to calm you down, help you relax, or help you sleep? (Drugs like Valium, Xanax, Ativan, Klonopin, Ambien, Sonata, or Lunesta?) **IF YES, specific drug(s) used:** _____	YES	NO	**E15**
E16	**Cannabis:** In the past 12 months, have you used marijuana ("pot," "grass," "weed"), hashish ("hash"), THC, K2, or "spice?" **IF YES, specific drug(s) used:** _____	YES	NO	**E16**
E17	**Stimulants:** In the past 12 months, have you used any stimulants or "uppers" to give you more energy, keep you alert, lose weight, or help you focus? (Drugs like speed, methamphetamine, crystal meth, "crank," Ritalin or methylphenidate, Dexedrine, Adderall or amphetamine, or prescription diet pills?) How about cocaine or "crack"? **IF YES, specific drug(s) used:** _____	YES	NO	**E17**
E18	**Opioids:** In the past 12 months, have you ever used heroin or methadone? How about prescription pain killers? (Drugs like morphine, codeine, Percocet, Percodan, Oxycontin, Tylox or oxycodone, Vicodin, Lortab, Lorcet or hydrocodone, Suboxone or buprenorphine?) **IF YES, specific drug(s) used:** _____	YES	NO	**E18**
E19	**Phencyclidine (PCP) and Related Substances:** In the past 12 months, have you ever used PCP ("angel dust," "peace pill") or ketamine ("Special K," "Vitamin K")? **IF YES, specific drug(s) used:** _____	YES	NO	**E19**
E20	**Other Hallucinogens:** In the past 12 months, have you used any drugs to "trip" or heighten your senses? (Drugs like LSD, "acid," peyote, mescaline, "mushrooms," psilocybin, Ecstasy [MDMA, "molly"], bath salts, DMT, or other hallucinogens?) **IF YES, specific drug(s) used:** _____	YES	NO	**E20**
E21	**Inhalants:** In the past 12 months, have you ever used glue, paint, correction fluid, gasoline, or other inhalants to get high? **IF YES, specific drug(s) used:** _____	YES	NO	**E21**
E22	**Other:** What about other drugs, like anabolic steroids, nitrous oxide (laughing gas, "whippets"), nitrites (amyl nitrite, butyl nitrite, "poppers," "snappers"), diet pills (phentermine), or over-the-counter medicine for allergies, colds, cough, or sleep? **IF YES, specific drug(s) used:** _____	YES	NO	**E22**

If <u>any</u> of items **E15–E22** have been rated "YES" (i.e., use of some substance in past 12 months), continue with the ratings for **E15a–E22a** on the **next page**.

If all of items **E15–E22** have been rated "NO," go to **F1** (Panic Disorder), **page 63**.

IF ACKNOWLEDGES USE OF A DRUG FROM ANY CLASS IN **E15–E22, page 56,** FOLLOW UP WITH THESE QUESTIONS TO DETERMINE WHETHER USE IS AT OR ABOVE THRESHOLD FOR ASSESSMENT OF SUBSTANCE USE DISORDER:

→ IF ILLICIT OR RECREATIONAL DRUG: **Have you used (SUBSTANCE) at least six times during the past 12 months?**

    IF YES: **During the past year, when were you taking (SUBSTANCE) the most? How long did that period last? During that time, how often were you taking it? How much were you using? Did your use of (SUBSTANCE) cause problems for you? Did anyone object to your use of (SUBSTANCE)?**

→ IF PRESCRIBED/OVER-THE-COUNTER (OTC) MEDICATION: **Over the past 12 months, did you get hooked or become dependent on (PRESCRIBED/OTC MEDICATION)? Did you ever take more of it than was prescribed or run out of your prescription early? Did you ever have to go to more than one doctor to make sure you didn't run out?**

	Drugs Used (recorded on page 56)	At or Above Assessment Threshold		Use Pattern (based on above questions)	
E15a	**Sedatives, Hypnotics, or Anxiolytics** Name of specific drug(s) used in this class:	YES	NO		E15a
E16a	**Cannabis** Name of specific drug(s) used in this class:	YES	NO		E16a
E17a	**Stimulants** Name of specific drug(s) used in this class:	YES	NO		E17a
E18a	**Opioids** Name of specific drug(s) used in this class:	YES	NO		E18a
E19a	**Phencyclidine and Related Substances** Name of specific drug(s) used in this class:	YES	NO		E19a
E20a	**Other Hallucinogens** Name of specific drug(s) used in this class:	YES	NO		E20a
E21a	**Inhalants** Name of specific drug(s) used in this class:	YES	NO		E21a
E22a	**Other** Name of specific drug(s) used in this class:	YES	NO		E22a

IF ANY CLASS OF ILLEGAL OR RECREATIONAL DRUGS WAS USED AT LEAST SIX TIMES WITHIN THE PAST 12 MONTHS OR PRESCRIBED/OTC MEDICATIONS WERE ABUSED OVER THE PAST 12 MONTHS (E.G., TAKING MORE THAN PRESCRIBED OR RECOMMENDED, DOCTOR SHOPPING TO GET PRESCRIPTIONS), GO TO **E23** (Past-12-Month Nonalcohol Substance Use Disorder), **page 58.**

OTHERWISE (I.E., NO DRUG USED AT LEAST SIX TIMES AND NO EVIDENCE OF PRESCRIPTION/OTC MEDICATION ABUSE), GO TO **F1** (Panic Disorder), **page 63.**

PAST-12-MONTH NONALCOHOL SUBSTANCE USE DISORDER	SUBSTANCE USE DISORDER CRITERIA			
E23	**I'd now like to ask you some more questions about your use of** (SUBSTANCE USED MOST HEAVILY OR CAUSED MOST PROBLEMS) **in the past 12 months, since** (ONE YEAR AGO).	A. A problematic pattern of substance use leading to clinically significant impairment or distress, as manifested by at least two of the following occurring within a 12-month period:			**E23**
E24	**During the past 12 months…** **…have you found that once you started using** (DRUG) **you ended up using much more than you <u>intended</u> to? For example, you planned to have** (SMALL AMOUNT OF DRUG) **but you ended up having much more. (Tell me about that. How often did that happen?)** IF NO: **What about using** (DRUG) **for a much longer period of time than you were <u>intending</u> to?**	1. The substance is often taken in larger amounts OR over a longer period than was intended.	—	+	**E24**
E25	**…have you wanted to stop or cut down using** (DRUG), **or control your use of** (DRUG)? ▶ IF YES: **How long did this desire to stop, cut down, or control your use of** (DRUG) **last?** ▶ IF NO: **During the past year, did you ever try to cut down, stop, or control your use of** (DRUG)? **How successful were you? (Did you make more than one attempt to stop, cut down, or control your use of** (DRUG)?**)**	2. There is a persistent desire OR unsuccessful efforts to cut down or control substance use.	—	+	**E25**
E26	**…have you spent a lot of time getting** (DRUG) **or using** (DRUG) **or has it taken a lot of time for you to get over the effects of** (DRUG)? **(How much time?)**	3. A great deal of time is spent in activities necessary to obtain the substance, use the substance, or recover from its effects.	—	+	**E26**
E27	**…have you had a strong desire or urge to use** (DRUG) **In between those times when you were using** (DRUG)? **(Has there been a time when you had such strong urges to use** (DRUG) **that you had trouble thinking about anything else?)** IF NO: **How about having a strong desire or urge to use** (DRUG) **when you were around people with whom you have used** (DRUG)?	4. Craving, or a strong desire or urge to use the substance.	—	+	**E27**

Which drugs or medications caused you the most problems over the past 12 months, since (ONE YEAR AGO)? **Which ones did you use the most? Which were your "drugs of choice"?**

E28	During the past 12 months, since (ONE YEAR AGO)...
	
	...have you missed work or school or often arrived late because you were intoxicated, high, or recovering from the night before?
	
	    IF NO: **How about doing a bad job at work or school, or failing courses or getting kicked out of school because of your use of** (DRUG)?
	
	        IF NO: **How about getting into trouble at work or school because of your use of** (DRUG)?
	
	            IF NO: **How about not taking care of things at home because of your use of** (DRUG), **like making sure there are food and clean clothes for your family and making sure your children go to school and get medical care? How about not paying your bills?**
	
	IF YES TO ANY: **How often?**
		5. Recurrent substance use resulting in a failure to fulfill major role obligations at work, school, or home (e.g., repeated absences or poor work performance related to substance use; substance-related absences, suspensions, or expulsions from school; neglect of children or household).	− +	E2

E29	...has your use of (DRUG) caused problems with other people, such as with family members, friends, or people at work? (**Have you found yourself regularly getting into arguments about your [DRUG] use? Have you gotten into physical fights when you were taking [DRUG]?**) IF YES: **Did you keep on using** (DRUG) **anyway? (Over what period of time?)**	6. Continued substance use despite having persistent or recurrent social or interpersonal problems caused or exacerbated by the effects of the substance (e.g., arguments with spouse about consequences of intoxication, physical fights).	− +	E2
E30	...have you had to give up or reduce the time you spent at work, with family or friends, or on your hobbies because you were using (DRUG) instead?	7. Important social, occupational, or recreational activities given up or reduced because of substance use.	− +	E3

E31	...have you ever gotten high before doing something that requires coordination and concentration like driving, boating, climbing on a ladder, or operating heavy machinery?
	
	    ▶ IF YES (FOR SUBSTANCES OTHER THAN STIMULANTS): **Would you say that your use of** (DRUG) **affected your coordination or concentration so that it was more likely that you or someone else could have been hurt?**
	
	    ▶ IF YES (FOR STIMULANTS ONLY): **Would you say that your being high on** (STIMULANT DRUG) **made you drive recklessly like driving very fast or taking unnecessary risks?**
	
	IF YES TO EITHER OF ABOVE AND IF UNKNOWN: **How many times?**
		8. Recurrent substance use in situations in which it is physically hazardous (e.g., driving an automobile or operating a machine when impaired by substance use).	− +	E3

E32	**During the past 12 months, since** (ONE YEAR AGO)… …**has your use of** (DRUG) **caused you any problems like making you very depressed, anxious, paranoid, very irritable, or extremely agitated? What about triggering panic attacks, making it difficult for you to sleep, putting you into a "mental fog," or making it so you couldn't recall what happened while you were using** (DRUG)**?** **Has your use of** (DRUG) **ever caused physical problems, like heart palpitations, coughing or trouble breathing, constipation, or skin infections?** IF YES TO EITHER OF ABOVE: **Did you keep on using** (DRUG) **anyway?**	9. Substance use is continued despite knowledge of having a persistent or recurrent physical or psychological problem that is likely to have been caused or exacerbated by the substance (e.g., recurrent cocaine use despite recognition of cocaine-related depression).	— +	**E32**
E33	…**have you found that you needed to use much more** (DRUG) **in order to get the feeling you wanted than when you first started using it?** ➤ IF YES: **How much more?** ➤ IF NO: **What about finding that when you used the same amount, it had much less effect than before?** IF PRESCRIBED MEDICATION: **Were you taking** (DRUG) **exactly as your doctor told you to? (Did you ever take more of it than was prescribed or run out of your prescription early? Did you ever go to more than one doctor in order to get the amount of medication you wanted?)**	10. Tolerance, as defined by either of the following: a. A need for markedly increased amounts of the substance to achieve intoxication or desired effect. b. Markedly diminished effect with continued use of the same amount of the substance.	— +	**E33**
E34	THE FOLLOWING ITEM DOES NOT APPLY TO PCP, HALLUCINOGENS, AND INHALANTS. **Have you ever had any withdrawal symptoms, in other words felt sick when you cut down or stopped using** (DRUG)**?** ➤ IF YES: **What symptoms did you have?** *(Refer to List of Withdrawal Symptoms on **page 62**.)* ➤ IF NO: **After not using** (DRUG) **for a few hours or more, did you sometimes use it or something like it to keep yourself from getting sick with** (WITHDRAWAL SYMPTOMS)**?** IF PRESCRIBED MEDICATION: **Were you taking this exactly as your doctor told you to? (Did you ever take more of it than was prescribed or run out of your prescription early? Did you ever have to go to more than one doctor to make sure you didn't run out?)**	11. Withdrawal, as manifested by either of the following: a. The characteristic withdrawal syndrome for the substance [see **page 62**]. b. The same (or a closely related) substance is taken to relieve or avoid withdrawal symptoms. *NOTE: This criterion applies to use of the following: sedatives, hypnotics, or anxiolytics; cannabis; stimulants/cocaine; and opioids. As in DSM-5, this criterion does not apply to PCP, hallucinogens, or inhalants.* *NOTE: This criterion is not considered met for individuals taking opioids; sedatives, hypnotics, or anxiolytics; or stimulant medications solely under medical supervision.*	— +	**E34**
E35	IF UNCLEAR: **When did** (ABOVE CRITERION A SXS [E24–E34] RATED "+") **occur? (Did they all happen within the past 12 months?)**	AT LEAST TWO OF THE ABOVE SUBSTANCE USE CRITERION A SXS **(E24–E34)** ARE RATED "+" AND SXS OCCURRED WITHIN THE PAST 12 MONTHS.	NO YES ↓ ↓	**E35**

If there is threshold use of other drug classes in past year (six or more times in 12 months or prescription abuse), return to **E23** on **page 58** and reassess the criteria for each drug class used at threshold in sequence until either criteria are met for a Substance Use Disorder in the past 12 months or else none of the drug classes meet criteria. If no drug class ultimately meets criteria, continue with **F1** (Panic Disorder), **page 63**.

Continue with **E36, next page.**

E36

<u>Diagnose</u> based on drug class and number of symptoms; indicate the diagnosis by circling the specific substance use disorder and severity level below:

E36

Sedative, Hypnotic, or Anxiolytic Use Disorder
  Mild: If 2–3 symptoms
  Moderate: If 4–5 symptoms
  Severe: If 6 or more symptoms

Specific drug used: _____

Cannabis Use Disorder
  Mild: If 2–3 symptoms
  Moderate: If 4–5 symptoms
  Severe: If 6 or more symptoms

Specific drug used: _____

Stimulant Use Disorder
    (including amphetamines, cocaine, and other stimulants)
  Mild: If 2–3 symptoms
  Moderate: If 4–5 symptoms
  Severe: If 6 or more symptoms

Specific drug used: _____

Opioid Use Disorder
  Mild: If 2–3 symptoms
  Moderate: If 4–5 symptoms
  Severe: If 6 or more symptoms

Specific drug used: _____

Phencyclidine and Related Substance Use Disorder
  Mild: If 2–3 symptoms
  Moderate: If 4–5 symptoms
  Severe: If 6 or more symptoms

Specific drug used: _____

Other Hallucinogen Use Disorder
  Mild: If 2–3 symptoms
  Moderate: If 4–5 symptoms
  Severe: If 6 or more symptoms

Specific drug used: _____

Inhalant Use Disorder
  Mild: If 2–3 symptoms
  Moderate: If 4–5 symptoms
  Severe: If 6 or more symptoms

Specific drug used: _____

Other (or Unknown) Substance Use Disorder
  Mild: If 2–3 symptoms
  Moderate: If 4–5 symptoms
  Severe: If 6 or more symptoms

Specific drug used: _____

List of Withdrawal Symptoms (from DSM-5 criteria for specific substance withdrawal diagnoses)

Listed below are the characteristic withdrawal syndromes for those classes of psychoactive substances for which a withdrawal syndrome has been identified. *(NOTE: A specific withdrawal syndrome has not been identified for PCP, HALLUCINOGENS, and INHALANTS.)* Withdrawal symptoms may occur following the cessation of prolonged moderate or heavy use of a psychoactive substance or a reduction in the amount used.

SEDATIVES, HYPNOTICS, OR ANXIOLYTICS

Two (or more) of the following, developing within several hours to a few days after the cessation of (or reduction in) sedative, hypnotic, or anxiolytic use that has been heavy and prolonged:

1. Autonomic hyperactivity (e.g., sweating or pulse rate greater than 100 bpm).
2. Hand tremor.
3. Insomnia.
4. Nausea or vomiting.
5. Transient visual, tactile, or auditory hallucinations or illusions.
6. Psychomotor agitation.
7. Anxiety.
8. Grand mal seizures.

CANNABIS

Three (or more) of the following signs and symptoms developing within approximately 1 week after cessation of cannabis use that has been heavy and prolonged (i.e., usually daily or almost daily use over a period of at least a few months):

1. Irritability, anger, or aggression.
2. Nervousness or anxiety.
3. Sleep difficulty (e.g., insomnia, disturbing dreams).
4. Decreased appetite or weight loss.
5. Restlessness.
6. Depressed mood.
7. At least one of the following physical symptoms causing significant discomfort: abdominal pain, shakiness/tremors, sweating, fever, chills, or headache.

STIMULANTS/COCAINE

Dysphoric mood AND two (or more) of the following physiological changes, developing within a few hours to several days after cessation of (or reduction in) prolonged amphetamine-type substance, cocaine, or other stimulant use:

1. Fatigue.
2. Vivid, unpleasant dreams.
3. Insomnia or hypersomnia.
4. Increased appetite.
5. Psychomotor retardation or agitation.

OPIOIDS

Three (or more) of the following, developing within minutes to several days after cessation of (or reduction in) opioid use that has been heavy and prolonged (i.e., several weeks or longer) or after administration of an opioid antagonist after a period of opioid use:

1. Dysphoric mood.
2. Nausea or vomiting.
3. Muscle aches.
4. Lacrimation or rhinorrhea (runny nose).
5. Pupillary dilation, piloerection [("goose bumps")], or sweating.
6. Diarrhea.
7. Yawning.
8. Fever.
9. Insomnia.

F. ANXIETY DISORDERS

	LIFETIME PANIC DISORDER	PANIC DISORDER CRITERIA		
F1	Have you ever had an intense rush of anxiety, or what someone might call a "panic attack," when you <u>suddenly</u> felt very frightened or anxious or suddenly developed a lot of physical symptoms? (Tell me about that.) When was the last bad one? What was it like? How did it begin? IF UNCLEAR: **Did the symptoms come on suddenly?** IF YES: **How long did it take from when it began to when it got really bad? (Did it happen within a few minutes?)**	A. [Panic Attack] A panic attack is an abrupt surge of intense fear or intense discomfort that reaches a peak within minutes, and during which time four (or more) of the following symptoms occur: **Note:** The abrupt surge can occur from a calm state or an anxious state.	— + Go to **F23** (Agoraphobia), **page 66.**	F
F2	During that attack… …did your heart race, pound, or skip?	1. Palpitations, pounding heart, or accelerated heart rate.	— +	F
F3	…did you sweat?	2. Sweating.	— +	F
F4	…did you tremble or shake?	3. Trembling or shaking.	— +	F
F5	…were you short of breath? (Have trouble catching your breath? Feel like you were being smothered?)	4. Sensations of shortness of breath or smothering.	— +	F
F6	…did you feel as if you were choking?	5. Feelings of choking.	— +	F
F7	…did you have chest pain or pressure?	6. Chest pain or discomfort.	— +	F
F8	…did you have nausea or upset stomach or the feeling that you were going to have diarrhea?	7. Nausea or abdominal distress.	— +	F
F9	…did you feel dizzy, unsteady, or like you might pass out?	8. Feeling dizzy, unsteady, light-headed, or faint.	— +	F
F10	…did you have flushes, hot flashes, or chills?	9. Chills or heat sensations.	— +	F
F11	…did you have tingling or numbness in parts of your body?	10. Paresthesias (numbness or tingling sensations).	— +	F

F12	...did you have the feeling that you were detached from your body or mind, that time was moving slowly, or that you were an outside observer of your own thoughts or movements?	11. Derealization (feelings of unreality) or depersonalization (being detached from oneself).	— +	F12
	IF NO: How about feeling that everything around you was unreal or that you were in a dream?			
F13	...were you afraid you were going crazy or might lose control?	12. Fear of losing control or "going crazy."	— +	F13
F14	...were you afraid that you were dying?	13. Fear of dying.	— +	F14
F15		AT LEAST FOUR OF THE ABOVE CRITERION A SXS (F2–F14) ARE RATED "+".	NO YES	F15

Besides the one you just described, have you had any other attacks which had even more of the symptoms that I just asked you about?

> IF YES: Go back to F2, page 63, and assess the symptoms for that attack.

> IF NO: Go to F23 (Agoraphobia), page 66.

Continue with F16, below.

F16	Have any of these attacks ever come on out of the blue—in situations where you didn't expect to be nervous or uncomfortable?	A. Recurrent unexpected panic attacks.	— +	F16
	IF YES: What was going on when the attack(s) happened? (What were you doing at the time? Were you already nervous or anxious at the time or rather were you relatively calm or relaxed?) How many of these kinds of attacks have you had? (At least two?)		Go to F23 (Agoraphobia), page 66.	
	IF NO: How about the very first one you had. What was going on in your life at that time? What were you doing at the time? Were you already nervous or anxious at the time or rather were you relatively calm or relaxed?)			
	IF ATTACK IS UNEXPECTED: How many of these kinds of attacks have you had? (At least two?)			
	After any of these attacks...	B. At least one of the attacks has been followed by 1 month (or more) of one or both of the following:		
F17	...were you concerned or worried that you might have another attack or worried that you would feel like you were having a heart attack again, or worried that you would lose control or go crazy?	1. Persistent concern or worry about additional panic attacks or their consequences (e.g., losing control, having a heart attack, "going crazy").	— +	F17
	IF YES: How long did that concern or worry last? (Did it last at least 1 month? Nearly every day?)			

F18	...**did you do anything differently because of the attacks (like avoiding certain places or not going out alone)? (What about avoiding certain activities like exercise? What about things like always making sure you're near a bathroom or exit?)** IF YES: **How long did that last? (As long as 1 month?)**	2. A significant maladaptive change in behavior related to the attacks (e.g., behaviors designed to avoid having panic attacks, such as avoidance of exercise or unfamiliar situations).	− +	F1
F19		CRITERION B1 **(F17)** OR B2 **(F18)** RATED "+". Go to **F23** (Agoraphobia), **page 66.**	NO YES ↓	F1
F20	IF UNKNOWN: **When did your panic attacks start?** **Just before you began having panic attacks, were you taking any drugs, caffeine, diet pills, or other medicines?** **(How much coffee, tea, or caffeinated beverages do you drink a day?)** **Just before the attacks, were you physically ill?** IF YES: **What did the doctor say?** Refer to the User's Guide, Section 9, for guidance on determining whether there is an etiological GMC or substance/medication.	C. [Primary Anxiety Disorder] The disturbance is not attributable to the physiological effects of a substance (e.g., a drug of abuse, a medication) or another medical condition (e.g., hypothyroidism, cardiopulmonary disorders). Etiological GMCs include endocrine disease (e.g., hyperthyroidism, pheochromocytoma, hypoglycemia, hyperadrenocortisolism), cardiovascular disorders (e.g., congestive heart failure, pulmonary embolism, arrhythmia such as atrial fibrillation), respiratory illness (e.g., chronic obstructive pulmonary disease, asthma, pneumonia), metabolic disturbances (e.g., vitamin B12 deficiency, porphyria), and neurological illness (e.g., neoplasms, vestibular dysfunction, encephalitis, seizure disorders). Etiological substances/medications include alcohol (I/W); caffeine (I); cannabis (I); opioids (W); phencyclidine (I); other hallucinogens (I); inhalants (I); stimulants (including cocaine) (I/W); sedatives, hypnotics, and anxiolytics (W); anesthetics and analgesics; sympathomimetics or other bronchodilators; anticholinergics; insulin; thyroid preparations; oral contraceptives; antihistamines; antiparkinsonian medications; corticosteroids; antihypertensive and cardiovascular medications; anticonvulsants; lithium carbonate; antipsychotic medications; antidepressant medications; and exposure to heavy metals and toxins such as organophosphate insecticide, nerve gases, carbon monoxide, carbon dioxide, and volatile substances such as gasoline and paint.	NO YES PRIMARY **Diagnose: Anxiety Disorder Due to AMC or Substance-Induced Anxiety Disorder;** Go to **F23** (Agoraphobia), **page 66.** Continue with **F21** (Criterion D), **below.**	F2
F21		D. The disturbance is not better explained by another mental disorder (e.g., the panic attacks do not occur only in response to feared social situations, as in Social Anxiety Disorder; in response to circumscribed phobic objects or situations, as in Specific Phobia; in response to obsessions, as in Obsessive-Compulsive Disorder; in response to reminders of traumatic events, as in Posttraumatic Stress Disorder; or in response to separation from attachment figures, as in Separation Anxiety Disorder).	NO YES ↓ Go to **F23** (Agoraphobia), **page 66.**	F2

| F22 | During the past month, since (ONE MONTH AGO), **how many panic attacks have you had?**

During the past month, **have you been concerned or worried that you might have another attack or worried that you would feel like you were having a heart attack again, or worried that you would lose control or go crazy?**

Have you done anything differently because of the attacks (like avoiding certain places or not going out alone)? | [During the past month, recurrent panic attacks (unexpected or expected) AND at least one of the attacks have been followed by persistent concern or worry about additional attacks or their consequences or a significant maladaptive change in behavior related to the attacks throughout the month.]

NO   **YES**
↓   ↓
Past Hx   Current
↓   ↓
Diagnose: Panic Disorder. Continue with **F23** (Agoraphobia), **below.** | F22 |

	CURRENT AGORAPHOBIA (PAST 6 MONTHS)	**AGORAPHOBIA CRITERIA**	
F23	**In the past 6 months, since** (6 MONTHS AGO), **have you been very anxious about or afraid of situations like going out of the house alone, being in crowds, going to stores, standing in lines, or traveling on buses or trains?** **Tell me about the situations that you've been afraid of.** IF UNKNOWN: **Have you been afraid of, or anxious about, traveling in taxicabs, buses, trains, ships or planes?** IF UNKNOWN: **How about being in open spaces, like parking lots, outdoor marketplaces, or bridges?** IF UNKNOWN: **How about being in enclosed places like stores, movie theaters, or shopping malls?** IF UNKNOWN: **How about standing in a line or being in a crowd?** IF UNKNOWN: **How about being outside of the house alone?**	A. Marked fear or anxiety about two (or more) of the following five situations: 1. Using public transportation (e.g., automobiles, buses, trains, ships, planes). 2. Being in open spaces (e.g., parking lots, marketplaces, bridges). 3. Being in enclosed places (e.g., shops, theaters, cinemas). 4. Standing in line or being in a crowd. 5. Being outside of the home alone.	F23
		— + ↓ Go to **F32** (Social Anxiety Disorder), **page 68.**	
F24	**Why have you been avoiding** (AVOIDED SITUATIONS) **or what have you been afraid would happen?** **(Have you been afraid that it might be hard for you to get out of** [AVOIDED SITUATIONS] **if you absolutely needed to...like if you suddenly developed a panic attack?)** **(Or developing something else that would be embarrassing like losing control of your bladder or bowels or vomiting?)** **(Have you been afraid of becoming impaired in some way, like by falling or passing out?)** **(How about being worried that there would be nobody there to help you in case these kinds of things happened?)**	B. The individual fears or avoids these situations because of thoughts that escape might be difficult or help might not be available in the event of developing panic-like symptoms or other incapacitating or embarrassing symptoms (e.g., fear of falling in the elderly, fear of incontinence).	F24
		— + ↓ Go to **F32** (Social Anxiety Disorder), **page 68.**	
F25	**Do you almost always feel frightened or anxious when you are in** (AVOIDED SITUATIONS)?	C. The agoraphobic situations almost always provoke fear or anxiety.	F25
		— + ↓ Go to **F32** (Social Anxiety Disorder), **page 68.**	

F26	Have you gone out of your way to avoid these situations? IF NO: **Have you been only able to go into one of these situations if you are with someone you know?** IF NO: **When you have had to be in one of these situations, have you felt intensely afraid or anxious?**	D. The agoraphobic situations are actively avoided, require the presence of a companion, or are endured with intense fear or anxiety.	— + ↓ Go to **F32** (Social Anxiety Disorder), **page 68.**	**F2**
F27	IF UNKNOWN: **Do you feel any danger or threat to your safety when you are in** (SITUATIONS)?	E. The fear or anxiety is out of proportion to the actual danger posed by the agoraphobic situations and to the sociocultural context.	— + ↓ Go to **F32** (Social Anxiety Disorder), **page 68.**	**F2**
F28	Has your fear or avoidance of (AVOIDED SITUATIONS) **been present for most of the past 6 months?**	F. The fear, anxiety, or avoidance is persistent, typically lasting for 6 months or more.	— + ↓ Go to **F32** (Social Anxiety Disorder), **page 68.**	**F2**
F29	IF UNCLEAR: **What effect have** (AGORAPHOBIC SXS) **had on your life?** ASK THE FOLLOWING QUESTIONS <u>ONLY AS NEEDED</u>: **How have** (AGORAPHOBIC SXS) **affected your relationships or your interactions with other people?** **(Have** [AGORAPHOBIC SXS] **caused any problems in your relationships with your family, romantic partner, or friends?)** **How have** (AGORAPHOBIC SXS) **affected your ability to work, take care of your family or household needs, or be involved in things that are important to you, like religious activities, physical exercise, or hobbies?** **Have** (AGORAPHOBIC SXS) **affected any other important part of your life?** IF AGORAPHOBIC SXS HAVE NOT INTERFERED WITH FUNCTIONING: **How much have you been bothered or upset by having** (AGORAPHOBIC SXS)**?**	G. The fear, anxiety, or avoidance causes clinically significant distress or impairment in social, occupational, or other important areas of functioning.	— + ↓ Go to **F32** (Social Anxiety Disorder), **page 68.**	**F2**
F30	IF A GMC CHARACTERIZED BY INCAPACITATING SYMPTOMS IS PRESENT: **Is your avoidance of** (AVOIDED SITUATION) **related to your** (MEDICAL CONDITION)? **(Tell me about it. How often has** [INCAPACITATING SYMPTOM] **actually happened in** [AVOIDED SITUATION]?**)**	H. If another medical condition (e.g., inflammatory bowel disease, Parkinson's disease) is present, the fear, anxiety, or avoidance is clearly excessive.	— + ↓ Go to **F32** (Social Anxiety Disorder), **page 68.**	**F3**

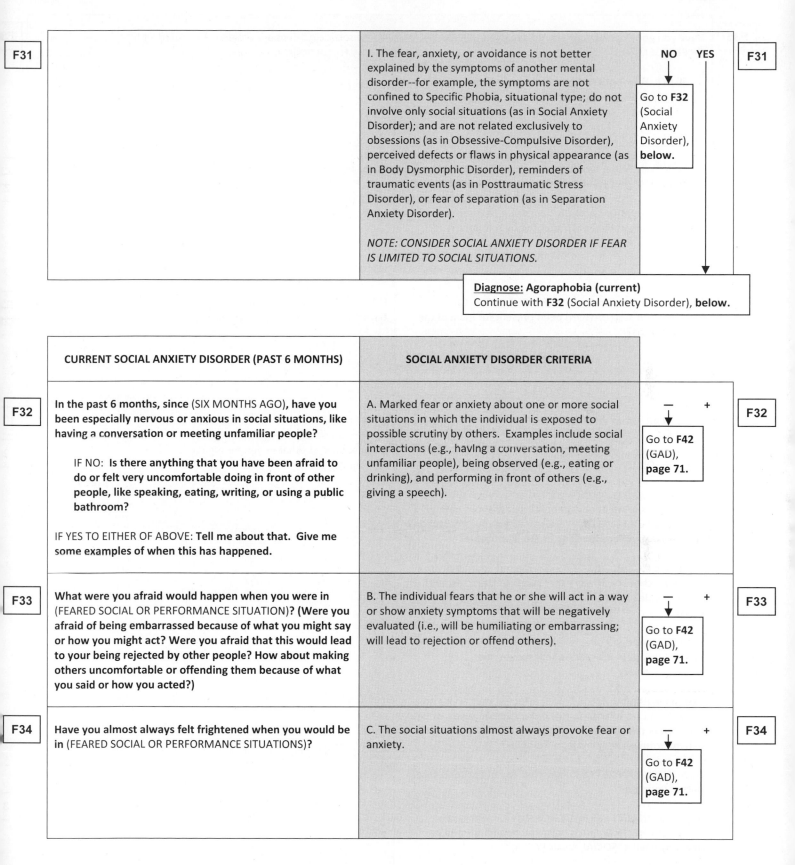

F31   I. The fear, anxiety, or avoidance is not better explained by the symptoms of another mental disorder--for example, the symptoms are not confined to Specific Phobia, situational type; do not involve only social situations (as in Social Anxiety Disorder); and are not related exclusively to obsessions (as in Obsessive-Compulsive Disorder), perceived defects or flaws in physical appearance (as in Body Dysmorphic Disorder), reminders of traumatic events (as in Posttraumatic Stress Disorder), or fear of separation (as in Separation Anxiety Disorder).

NO   YES

Go to **F32** (Social Anxiety Disorder), **below.**

F31

NOTE: CONSIDER SOCIAL ANXIETY DISORDER IF FEAR IS LIMITED TO SOCIAL SITUATIONS.

<u>Diagnose:</u> **Agoraphobia (current)**
Continue with **F32** (Social Anxiety Disorder), **below.**

CURRENT SOCIAL ANXIETY DISORDER (PAST 6 MONTHS)	SOCIAL ANXIETY DISORDER CRITERIA	
F32 In the past 6 months, since (SIX MONTHS AGO), have you been especially nervous or anxious in social situations, like having a conversation or meeting unfamiliar people? IF NO: Is there anything that you have been afraid to do or felt very uncomfortable doing in front of other people, like speaking, eating, writing, or using a public bathroom? IF YES TO EITHER OF ABOVE: Tell me about that. Give me some examples of when this has happened.	A. Marked fear or anxiety about one or more social situations in which the individual is exposed to possible scrutiny by others. Examples include social interactions (e.g., having a conversation, meeting unfamiliar people), being observed (e.g., eating or drinking), and performing in front of others (e.g., giving a speech).	− + ↓ Go to **F42** (GAD), **page 71.** **F32**
F33 What were you afraid would happen when you were in (FEARED SOCIAL OR PERFORMANCE SITUATION)? (Were you afraid of being embarrassed because of what you might say or how you might act? Were you afraid that this would lead to your being rejected by other people? How about making others uncomfortable or offending them because of what you said or how you acted?)	B. The individual fears that he or she will act in a way or show anxiety symptoms that will be negatively evaluated (i.e., will be humiliating or embarrassing; will lead to rejection or offend others).	− + ↓ Go to **F42** (GAD), **page 71.** **F33**
F34 Have you almost always felt frightened when you would be in (FEARED SOCIAL OR PERFORMANCE SITUATIONS)?	C. The social situations almost always provoke fear or anxiety.	− + ↓ Go to **F42** (GAD), **page 71.** **F34**

F35	**Have you gone out of your way to avoid** (FEARED SOCIAL OR PERFORMANCE SITUATION)? IF NO: **How hard is it for you to be in** (FEARED SOCIAL OR PERFORMANCE SITUATION)?	D. The social situations are avoided or endured with intense fear or anxiety.	— + ↓ Go to **F42** (GAD), **page 71.** **F3**
F36	IF UNKNOWN: **What would you say would be the likely outcome of** (PERFORMING POORLY IN SOCIAL SITUATION)? **(Are these situations actually dangerous in some way, like avoiding being bullied or tormented by someone?)**	E. The fear or anxiety is out of proportion to the actual threat posed by the social situation and to the sociocultural context.	— + ↓ Go to **F42** (GAD), **page 71.** **F3**
F37	**Has your fear or avoidance of** (FEARED SOCIAL OR PERFORMANCE SITUATION) **been present for most of the past 6 months?**	F. The fear, anxiety, or avoidance is persistent, typically lasting for 6 months or more.	— + ↓ Go to **F42** (GAD), **page 71.** **F3**
F38	IF UNCLEAR: **What effect have** (SOCIAL ANXIETY SXS) **had on your life?** ASK THE FOLLOWING QUESTIONS <u>ONLY AS NEEDED</u>: **How have** (SOCIAL ANXIETY SXS) **affected your ability to have friends or meet new people? (How about dating?)** **How have** (SOCIAL ANXIETY SXS) **affected your interactions with other people, especially unfamiliar people?** **How have** (SOCIAL ANXIETY SXS) **affected your ability to do things at school or at work that require interacting with other people? How about making presentations or giving talks?** **Have you avoided going to school or to work if you think you will be put in a situation that makes your uncomfortable?** **How have** (SOCIAL ANXIETY SXS) **affected your ability to work, take care of your family or household needs, or be involved in things that are important to you, like religious activities, physical exercise, or hobbies?** **Have** (SOCIAL ANXIETY SXS) **affected any other important part of your life?** IF SOCIAL ANXIETY SXS HAVE NOT INTERFERED WITH FUNCTIONING: **How much have you been bothered or upset by having** (SOCIAL ANXIETY SXS)?	G. The fear, anxiety, or avoidance causes clinically significant distress or impairment in social, occupational, or other important areas of functioning.	— + ↓ Go to **F42** (GAD), **page 71.** **F3**

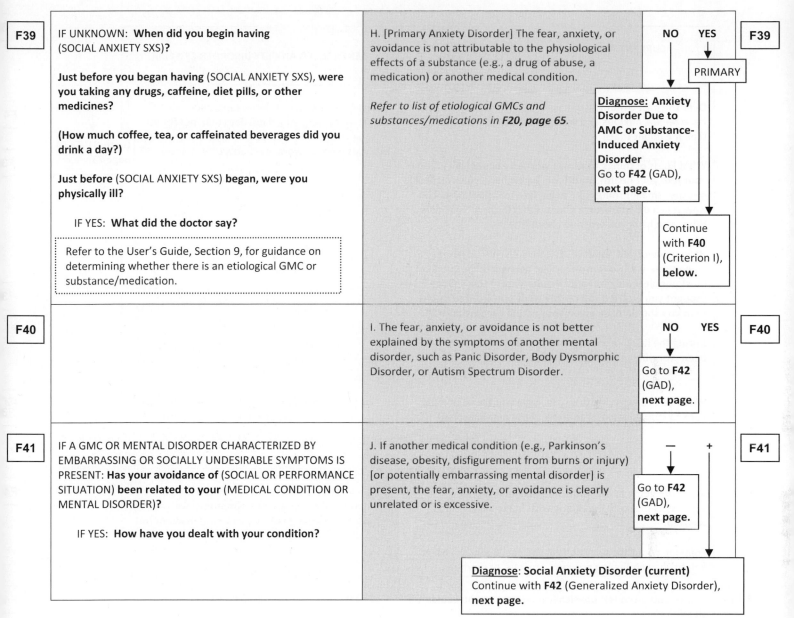

F39

IF UNKNOWN: **When did you begin having** (SOCIAL ANXIETY SXS)**?**

Just before you began having (SOCIAL ANXIETY SXS)**, were you taking any drugs, caffeine, diet pills, or other medicines?**

(**How much coffee, tea, or caffeinated beverages did you drink a day?**)

Just before (SOCIAL ANXIETY SXS) **began, were you physically ill?**

   IF YES: **What did the doctor say?**

Refer to the User's Guide, Section 9, for guidance on determining whether there is an etiological GMC or substance/medication.

H. [Primary Anxiety Disorder] The fear, anxiety, or avoidance is not attributable to the physiological effects of a substance (e.g., a drug of abuse, a medication) or another medical condition.

Refer to list of etiological GMCs and substances/medications in F20, page 65.

NO   YES   **F39**

PRIMARY

Diagnose: Anxiety Disorder Due to AMC or Substance-Induced Anxiety Disorder Go to **F42** (GAD), **next page.**

Continue with **F40** (Criterion I), **below.**

F40

I. The fear, anxiety, or avoidance is not better explained by the symptoms of another mental disorder, such as Panic Disorder, Body Dysmorphic Disorder, or Autism Spectrum Disorder.

NO   YES   **F40**

Go to **F42** (GAD), **next page.**

F41

IF A GMC OR MENTAL DISORDER CHARACTERIZED BY EMBARRASSING OR SOCIALLY UNDESIRABLE SYMPTOMS IS PRESENT: **Has your avoidance of** (SOCIAL OR PERFORMANCE SITUATION) **been related to your** (MEDICAL CONDITION OR MENTAL DISORDER)**?**

   IF YES: **How have you dealt with your condition?**

J. If another medical condition (e.g., Parkinson's disease, obesity, disfigurement from burns or injury) [or potentially embarrassing mental disorder] is present, the fear, anxiety, or avoidance is clearly unrelated or is excessive.

—   +   **F41**

Go to **F42** (GAD), **next page.**

Diagnose: **Social Anxiety Disorder (current)** Continue with **F42** (Generalized Anxiety Disorder), **next page.**

	CURRENT GENERALIZED ANXIETY DISORDER (PAST 6 MONTHS)	GENERALIZED ANXIETY DISORDER CRITERIA		
F42	Over the past 6 months, since (6 MONTHS AGO), have you been feeling anxious and worried for a lot of the time? (Tell me about that.) What kinds of things have you worried about? (What about your job, your health, your family members, your finances, or other smaller things like being late for appointments?) How much did you worry about (EVENTS OR ACTIVITIES)? What else have you worried about? Have you worried about (EVENTS OR ACTIVITIES) **even when there was no reason? (Have you worried more than most people would in your circumstances? Has anyone else thought you worried too much? Have you worried more than you should have given your actual circumstances?)** During the last 6 months, would you say that you have been worrying more days than not?	A. Excessive anxiety and worry (apprehensive expectation), occurring more days than not for at least 6 months, about a number of events or activities (such as work or school performance).	− + ↓ Go to **G1** (OCD), page 73.	F4
F43	When you're worrying this way, have you found that it's hard to stop yourself or to think about anything else?	B. The individual finds it difficult to control the worry.	− + ↓ Go to **G1** (OCD), page 73.	F4
F44	Now I am going to ask you some questions about symptoms that often go along with being nervous or worried. Thinking about those periods in the past 6 months when you have been feeling nervous, anxious, or worried...	C. The anxiety and worry are associated with three (or more) of the following six symptoms (with at least some symptoms present for more days than not for the past 6 months):		F4
F45	...have you often felt physically restless, like you couldn't sit still? ...have you often felt keyed up or on edge?	1. Restlessness or feeling keyed up or on edge.	− +	F4
F46	...have you often tired easily?	2. Being easily fatigued.	− +	F4
F47	...have you often had trouble concentrating or has your mind often gone blank?	3. Difficulty concentrating or mind going blank.	− +	F4
F48	...have you often been irritable?	4. Irritability.	− +	F4
F49	...have your muscles often been tense?	5. Muscle tension.	− +	F4
F50	...have you often had trouble falling or staying asleep? How about often feeling tired when you woke up because you didn't get a good night's sleep?	6. Sleep disturbance (difficulty falling or staying asleep, or restless unsatisfying sleep).	− +	F5

F51		AT LEAST THREE OF THE ABOVE CRITERION C SXS **(F45–F50)** ARE RATED "+".　　　－　　＋ ↓ Go to **G1** (OCD), **page 73.**	**F51**

F52	IF UNCLEAR: **What effect have** (GAD SXS) **had on your life?** ASK THE FOLLOWING QUESTIONS <u>ONLY AS NEEDED</u>: **How have** (GAD SXS) **affected your relationships or your interactions with other people? (Have** [GAD SXS] **caused you any problems in your relationships with your family, romantic partner, or friends?)** **How have** (GAD SXS) **affected your work/schoolwork? (How about your attendance at work/school? Have** [GAD SXS] **made it more difficult to do your work/schoolwork? Have** [GAD SXS] **affected the quality of your work/schoolwork?)** **How have** (GAD SXS) **affected your ability to take care of things at home? How about doing other things that are important to you, like religious activities, physical exercise, or hobbies? Have you avoided doing anything because you felt like you weren't up to it?** **Has your anxiety or worry affected any other important part of your life?** IF DOES NOT INTERFERE WITH LIFE: **How much have you been bothered or upset by having** (GAD SXS)**?**	D. The anxiety, worry, or physical symptoms cause clinically significant distress or impairment in social, occupational, or other important areas of functioning.　　　－　　＋ ↓ Go to **G1** (OCD), **page 73.**	**F52**

F53	IF UNKNOWN: **When did your** (GAD SXS) **begin?** **Just before you began having** (GAD SXS), **were you taking any drugs, caffeine, diet pills, or other medicines? (How much coffee, tea, or caffeinated beverages did you drink a day?)** **Just before** (GAD SXS) **began, were you physically ill?** 　　IF YES: **What did the doctor say?** Refer to the User's Guide, Section 9, for guidance on determining whether there is an etiological GMC or substance/medication.	E. [Primary Anxiety Disorder] The disturbance is not attributable to the physiological effects of a substance (e.g., a drug of abuse, a medication) or another medical condition (e.g., hyperthyroidism). *Refer to list of etiological GMCs and substances/medications in F20, page 65.* NO　　YES ↓　　　PRIMARY <u>Diagnose:</u> **Anxiety Disorder Due to AMC or Substance-Induced Anxiety Disorder;** Go to **G1** (OCD), **next page.** Continue with **F54 below.**	**F53**

F54		F. The disturbance is not better explained by another mental disorder (e.g., anxiety or worry about having panic attacks in Panic Disorder, negative evaluation in Social Anxiety Disorder, contamination or other obsessions in Obsessive-Compulsive Disorder, separation from attachment figures in Separation Anxiety Disorder, reminders of traumatic events in Posttraumatic Stress Disorder, gaining weight in Anorexia Nervosa, physical complaints in Somatic Symptom Disorder, perceived appearance flaws in Body Dysmorphic Disorder, having a serious illness in Illness Anxiety Disorder, or the content of delusional beliefs in Schizophrenia or Delusional Disorder). NO　　YES ↓ Go to **G1** (OCD), **next page.**	**F54**

<u>Diagnose:</u> Generalized Anxiety Disorder (current).
Continue with **G1** (Obsessive-Compulsive Disorder), **next page.**

G. OBSESSIVE-COMPULSIVE DISORDER and POSTTRAUMATIC STRESS DISORDER

Obsessive-Compulsive Disorder

CURRENT OBSESSIVE-COMPULSIVE DISORDER	OBSESSIVE-COMPULSIVE DISORDER CRITERIA	
In the past month, since (ONE MONTH AGO)...	A. Presence of obsessions, compulsions, or both: Obsessions are defined by (1) and (2):	
G1 ...**have you been bothered by thoughts that kept coming back to you even when you didn't want them to, like being exposed to germs or dirt or needing everything to be lined up in a certain way? (What were they?)** **How about having urges to do something that kept coming back to you even though you didn't want them to, like an urge to harm a loved one? (What were they?)** **How about having images popping into your head that you didn't want, like violent or horrible scenes or something of a sexual nature? (What were they?)** IF YES TO ANY OF ABOVE: **Have these** (THOUGHTS/URGES/IMAGES) **made you very anxious or upset?**	1. Recurrent and persistent thoughts, urges, or images that are experienced, at some time during the disturbance, as intrusive and unwanted, and that in most individuals cause marked anxiety or distress.	— + ↓ Go to **G3** (Compulsions), below. **G1**
G2 **When you had these** (THOUGHTS/URGES/IMAGES) **did you try hard to get them out of your head? (What would you try to do?)**	2. The individual attempts to ignore or suppress such thoughts, urges, or images, or to neutralize them with some other thought or action (i.e., by performing a compulsion).	— + ↓ OBSESSIONS ↓ Go to **G3** (Compulsions), below. **G2**
In the past month, since (ONE MONTH AGO)...	Compulsions are defined by (1) and (2):	
G3 ...**was there anything that you had to do over and over again and was hard to resist doing, like washing your hands again and again, repeating something over and over again until it "felt right," counting up to a certain number, or checking something many times to make sure that you'd done it right?** **Tell me about that. (What did you have to do?)**	1. Repetitive behaviors (e.g., hand washing, ordering, checking) or mental acts (e.g., praying, counting, repeating words silently) that the individual feels driven to perform in response to an obsession or according to rules that must be applied rigidly.	— + ↓ Go to **G5**, next page. **G3**
G4 IF UNCLEAR: **Why did you have to do** (COMPULSIVE ACT)? **What would happen if you didn't do it?** IF UNCLEAR: **How many times would you do** (COMPULSIVE ACT)? **Are you doing** (COMPULSIVE ACT) **more than really makes sense?**	2. The behaviors or mental acts are aimed at preventing or reducing anxiety or distress, or preventing some dreaded event or situation; however, these behaviors or mental acts either are not connected in a realistic way with what they are designed to neutralize or prevent, or are clearly excessive.	— + ↓ COMPULSIONS ↓ Go to **G5**, next page. **G4**

G5	**CHECK FOR OBSESSIONS AND/OR COMPULSIONS**	PRESENCE OF OBSESSIONS (**G2** RATED "+") OR COMPULSIONS (**G4** RATED "+")	NO　　　YES ↓ Go to **G9** (PTSD), **page 76.**	G5
G6	IF UNCLEAR: **How much time have you spent on** (OBSESSION OR COMPULSION)? IF UNCLEAR: **What effect did this these** (OBSESSIONS OR COMPULSIONS) **have on your life?** ASK THE FOLLOWING QUESTIONS <u>ONLY AS NEEDED</u>: **How have** (OBSESSIONS OR COMPULSIONS) **affected your relationships or your interactions with other people? (Have** [OBSESSIONS OR COMPULSIONS] **caused you any problems in your relationships with your family, romantic partner, roommates, or friends?)** **How have** (OBSESSIONS OR COMPULSIONS) **affected your work/school? (How about your attendance at work/school? Have** [OBSESSIONS OR COMPULSIONS] **made it more difficult to do your work/schoolwork? Have** [OBSESSIONS OR COMPULSIONS] **affected the quality of your work/schoolwork?)** **How have** (OBSESSIONS OR COMPULSIONS) **affected your ability to take care of things at home? How about doing other things that are important to you, like religious activities, physical exercise, or hobbies?** **Have** (OBSESSIONS OR COMPULSIONS) **affected any other important part of your life?** IF HAVE NOT INTERFERED WITH LIFE: **How much have you been bothered by having** (OBSESSIONS OR COMPULSIONS)?	B. The obsessions or compulsions are time-consuming (e.g., take more than 1 hour per day) or cause clinically significant distress or impairment in social, occupational, or other important areas of functioning.	—　　　+ ↓ Go to **G9** (PTSD), **page 76.**	G6
G7	IF UNKNOWN: **When did** (OBSESSIONS OR COMPULSIONS) **begin?** **Just before you began having** (OBSESSIONS OR COMPULSIONS), **were you taking any drugs or medicines?** **Just before the** (OBSESSIONS OR COMPULSIONS) **started, were you physically ill?** 　IF YES: **What did the doctor say?** ┌┈┈┈┈┈┈┈┈┈┈┈┈┈┈┈┈┈┈┈┈┈┈┈┈┐ Refer to the User's Guide, Section 9, for guidance on determining whether there is an etiological GMC or substance/medication. └┈┈┈┈┈┈┈┈┈┈┈┈┈┈┈┈┈┈┈┈┈┈┈┈┘	C. [Primary Obsessive-Compulsive Disorder] The obsessive-compulsive symptoms are not attributable to the physiological effects of a substance (e.g., a drug of abuse, a medication) or another medical condition. <u>Etiological GMCs include</u> Sydenham's chorea and medical conditions leading to striatal damage, such as cerebral infarction. <u>Etiological substances/medications include</u> intoxication with cocaine, amphetamines, or other stimulants, and exposure to heavy metals.	NO　　　YES ↓　　　　↓ 　　　┌─────────┐ 　　　│ PRIMARY │ 　　　└─────────┘ ┌──────────────┐ **Diagnose: OC and Related Disorder Due to AMC or Substance-Induced OC and Related Disorder.** Go to **G9** (PTSD), **page 76.** └──────────────┘ ┌──────────────┐ Continue with **G8, next page.** └──────────────┘	G7

G8

D. The disturbance is not better explained by the symptoms of another mental disorder (e.g., excessive worries, as in Generalized Anxiety Disorder; preoccupation with appearance, as in Body Dysmorphic Disorder; difficulty discarding or parting with possessions, as in Hoarding Disorder; hair pulling, as in Trichotillomania [Hair-Pulling Disorder]; skin picking, as in Excoriation [Skin-Picking] Disorder; stereotypies, as in Stereotypic Movement Disorder; ritualized eating behavior, as in Eating Disorders; preoccupation with substances or gambling, as in Substance-Related and Addictive Disorders; preoccupation with having an illness, as in Illness Anxiety Disorder; sexual urges or fantasies, as in Paraphilic Disorders; impulses, as in Disruptive, Impulse-Control, and Conduct Disorders; guilty ruminations, as in Major Depressive Disorder; thought insertion or delusional preoccupations, as in Schizophrenia Spectrum and Other Psychotic Disorders; or repetitive patterns of behavior, as in Autism Spectrum Disorder).

NO   YES

Go to **G9** (PTSD), **next page.**

G8

Diagnose: **Obsessive-Compulsive Disorder (current).**
Continue with **G9** (PTSD), **next page.**

Posttraumatic Stress Disorder

G9

LIFETIME TRAUMA HISTORY

I'd now like to ask about some things that may have happened to you that may have been extremely upsetting. People often find that talking about these experiences can be helpful. I'll start by asking if these experiences apply to you, and If so, I'll ask you to briefly describe what happened and how you felt at the time.

SCREEN FOR EACH TYPE OF TRAUMA (BASED ON DSM-5 TEXT AND PTSD CRITERION A) USING THE QUESTIONS BELOW.
Have you ever been in a life-threatening situation like a major disaster or fire, combat, or a serious car or work-related accident?

What about being physically or sexually assaulted or abused, or threatened with physical or sexual assault?

How about seeing another person being physically or sexually assaulted or abused, or threatened with physical or sexual assault?

Have you ever seen another person killed or dead, or badly hurt?

How about learning that one of these things happened to someone you are close to?

IF UNKNOWN: **Have you ever been the victim of a serious crime?**

IF NO EVENTS ENDORSED: **What would you say has been the most stressful or traumatic experience you have had over your life?**

IF NO EVENTS ACKNOWLEDGED, CONTINUE WITH **H1** (Attention-Deficit/Hyperactivity Disorder), **page 86.**

IF ANY EVENTS ACKNOWLEDGED: IN **G10–G12** BELOW, REVIEW AND INQUIRE IN DETAIL FOR UP TO THREE PAST EVENTS (E.G., SELECT THREE WORST EVENTS; SELECT TRAUMA OF INTEREST PLUS TWO OTHER WORST EVENTS).

PAST LIFETIME EVENT #1:

G10

IF DIRECT EXPOSURE TO TRAUMA:
What happened? Were you afraid of dying or being seriously hurt? Were you seriously hurt?

IF WITNESSED TRAUMATIC EVENT HAPPENING TO OTHERS:
What happened? What did you see? How close were you to (TRAUMATIC EVENT)? Were you concerned about your own safety?

IF LEARNED ABOUT TRAUMATIC EVENT:
What happened? Who did it involve? (How close [emotionally] were you to them? Did it involve violence, suicide, or a bad accident?)

IF UNKNOWN: **How old were you at the time?**

IF UNKNOWN: **Did this happen more than once?**

Description of traumatic event:

Indicate type of traumatic event (check all that apply):
___Death, actual
___Death, threatened
___Serious injury, actual
___Serious injury, threatened
___Sexual violence, actual
___Sexual violence, threatened

Indicate mode of exposure to traumatic event:
___Directly experienced
___Witnessed happening to others in person
___Learning about event in close family member or friend
___Repeated or extreme exposure to aversive details of traumatic events (e.g., police officers repeatedly exposed to details of child abuse)

Age at time of event: _____

Indicate single event vs. prolonged/repeated exposure by circling appropriate number:
　　1—Single event
　　2—Prolonged or repeated exposure to same trauma (e.g., witnessing repeated episodes of parental domestic violence over years)

PAST LIFETIME EVENT #2:

G11

IF DIRECT EXPOSURE TO TRAUMA:
What happened? Were you afraid of dying or being seriously hurt? Were you seriously hurt?

IF WITNESSED TRAUMATIC EVENT HAPPENING TO OTHERS:
What happened? What did you see? How close were you to (TRAUMATIC EVENT)? Were you concerned about your own safety?

IF LEARNED ABOUT TRAUMATIC EVENT:
What happened? Who did it involve? (How close [emotionally] were you to them? Did it involve violence, suicide, or a bad accident?)

IF UNKNOWN: **How old were you at the time?**

IF UNKNOWN: **Did this happen more than once?**

Description of traumatic event:

Indicate type of traumatic event (check all that apply):
___ Death, actual
___ Death, threatened
___ Serious injury, actual
___ Serious injury, threatened
___ Sexual violence, actual
___ Sexual violence, threatened

Indicate mode of exposure to traumatic event:
___ Directly experienced
___ Witnessed happening to others in person
___ Learning about event in close family member or friend
___ Repeated or extreme exposure to aversive details of traumatic events (e.g., police officers repeatedly exposed to details of child abuse)

Age at time of event: _____

Indicate single event vs. prolonged/repeated exposure by circling appropriate number:
     1—Single event
     2—Prolonged or repeated exposure to same trauma (e.g., witnessing repeated episodes of parental domestic violence over years)

G11

PAST LIFETIME EVENT #3:

G12

IF DIRECT EXPOSURE TO TRAUMA:
What happened? Were you afraid of dying or being seriously hurt? Were you seriously hurt?

IF WITNESSED TRAUMATIC EVENT HAPPENING TO OTHERS:
What happened? What did you see? How close were you to (TRAUMATIC EVENT)? Were you concerned about your own safety?

IF LEARNED ABOUT TRAUMATIC EVENT:
What happened? Who did it involve? (How close [emotionally] were you to them? Did it involve violence, suicide, or a bad accident?)

IF UNKNOWN: **How old were you at the time?**

IF UNKNOWN: **Did this happen more than once?**

Description of traumatic event:

Indicate type of traumatic event (check all that apply):
___ Death, actual
___ Death, threatened
___ Serious injury, actual
___ Serious injury, threatened
___ Sexual violence, actual
___ Sexual violence, threatened

Indicate mode of exposure to traumatic event:
___ Directly experienced
___ Witnessed happening to others in person
___ Learning about event in close family member or friend
___ Repeated or extreme exposure to aversive details of traumatic events (e.g., police officers repeatedly exposed to details of child abuse)

Age at time of event: ___

Indicate single event vs. prolonged/repeated exposure by circling appropriate number:
     1—Single event
     2—Prolonged or repeated exposure to same trauma (e.g., witnessing repeated episodes of parental domestic violence over years)

G12

CURRENT POSTTRAUMATIC STRESS DISORDER	POSTTRAUMATIC STRESS DISORDER CRITERIA	
G13 IF THE ONLY EXPOSURE TO TRAUMA EVENTS HAS BEEN WITHIN THE PAST MONTH, GO TO **H1** (ADHD). IF MORE THAN ONE TRAUMATIC EVENT IS REPORTED: **Which of these** (EVENT FROM G10–G12) **do you think affected you the most?** PAST LIFETIME EVENT #_____ RATE **G13–G41** (ASSESSMENT OF PTSD CRITERIA) USING SELECTED EVENT ABOVE. AS NOTED IN **G19, G22, G30, G37, G38, G39, G40,** IF SELECTED EVENT IS NOT ASSOCIATED WITH FULL PTSD, CONSIDER REASSESSING THE ENTIRE PTSD CRITERIA SET **(G13–G41)** USING OTHER REPORTED TRAUMAS **(G10–G12).**	A. Exposure to actual or threatened death, serious injury, or sexual violence in one (or more) of the following ways: 1. Directly experiencing the traumatic event(s). 2. Witnessing, in person, the event(s) as it occurred to others. 3. Learning that the traumatic event(s) occurred to a close family member or close friend. In cases of actual or threatened death of a family member or friend, the event(s) must have been violent or accidental. 4. Experiencing repeated or extreme exposure to aversive details of the traumatic event(s) (e.g., first responders collecting human remains; police officers repeatedly exposed to details of child abuse). **Note:** Criterion A4 does not apply to exposure through electronic media, television, movies, or pictures, unless this exposure is work related.	– + **G13** ↓ Go to **H1** (ADHD), **page 86.**
Now I'd like to ask a few questions about specific ways that (TRAUMATIC EVENT) **may have affected you at any time since** (TRAUMATIC EVENT). **For example, since** (TRAUMATIC EVENT)...	B. Presence of one (or more) of the following intrusion symptoms associated with the traumatic event(s), beginning after the traumatic event(s) occurred:	
G14 ...**have you had memories of** (TRAUMATIC EVENT), **including feelings, physical sensations, sounds, smells, or images, when you didn't expect to or want to? (How often has this happened?)** IF LIFETIME RATING OF "+": **Has this also been the case in the past month, since** (ONE MONTH AGO)? **How many times?**	1. Recurrent, involuntary, and intrusive distressing memories of the traumatic event(s).	– + **G14** ↓ Past month – +
G15 ...**what about repeatedly having upsetting dreams that reminded you of** (TRAUMATIC EVENT)? **(Tell me about that.)** IF LIFETIME RATING OF "+": **Has this also happened in the past month? How many times?**	2. Recurrent distressing dreams in which the content and/or affect of the dream are related to the traumatic events.	– + **G15** ↓ Past month – +
G16 ...**what about having found yourself acting or feeling as if you were back in the situation? (Have you had "flashbacks" of** [TRAUMATIC EVENT]?) IF LIFETIME RATING OF "+": **Has this also happened in the past month? How many times?**	3. Dissociative reactions (e.g., flashbacks) in which the individual feels or acts as if the traumatic event(s) were recurring. (Such reactions may occur on a continuum, with the most extreme expression being a complete loss of awareness of present surroundings.)	– + **G16** ↓ Past month – +

Since (TRAUMATIC EVENT)...

...have you had a strong emotional or physical reaction when something reminded you of (TRAUMATIC EVENT)?

Give me some examples of the kinds of things that would have triggered this reaction. (Things like...seeing a person who resembles the person who attacked you, hearing the screech of brakes if you were in a car accident, hearing the sound of helicopters if you were in combat, any kind of physically intimacy if you were raped?)

NOTE: IF DENIES EMOTIONAL OR PHYSICAL REACTION TO REMINDERS, CODE "—" FOR BOTH **G17** (EMOTIONAL REACTION) AND **G18** (PHYSICAL REACTION).

G17	IF ACKNOWLEDGES STRONG EMOTIONAL OR PHYSICAL REACTION: **What kind of reaction did you have? Did you get very upset or stay upset for a while, even after the reminder had gone away?** IF LIFETIME RATING OF "+": **Has this also happened in the past month? How many times?**	4. Intense or prolonged psychological distress at exposure to internal or external cues that symbolize or resemble an aspect of the traumatic event(s).	— + ↓ Past month — +	G1
G18	IF ACKNOWLEDGES STRONG EMOTIONAL OR PHYSICAL REACTION: **What about having physical symptoms— like breaking out in a sweat, breathing heavily or irregularly, or feeling your heart pound or race when something reminded you of (TRAUMATIC EVENT)? How about feeling tense or shaky?** IF LIFETIME RATING OF "+": **Has this also happened in the past month? How many times?**	5. Marked physiological reactions to internal or external cues that symbolize or resemble an aspect of the traumatic event(s).	— + ↓ Past month — +	G1
G19		AT LEAST ONE OF THE ABOVE CRITERION B SXS **(G14–G18)** IS RATED "+". If other reported traumatic events, consider returning to **G13** and reassessing PTSD for that event. Otherwise, go to **H1** (ADHD), **page 86**.	NO YES ↓ Criterion B met past month. NO YES	G1

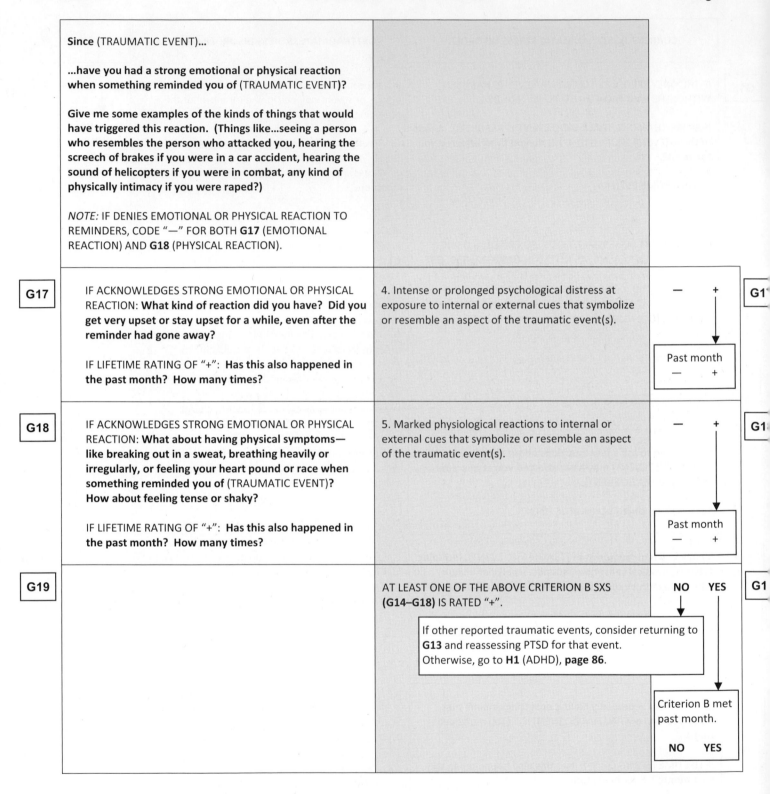

	C. Persistent avoidance of stimuli associated with the traumatic event(s), beginning after the traumatic event(s) occurred, as evidenced by one or both of the following:	

Since (TRAUMATIC EVENT)...

G20

...**have you done things to avoid remembering or thinking about** (TRAUMATIC EVENT), **like keeping yourself busy, distracting yourself by playing computer or video games or watching TV, or using drugs or alcohol to "numb" yourself or try to forget what happened? How long has this gone on? (Almost all of the time for more than 1 month?)**

   IF NO: **How about doing things to avoid having feelings similar to those you had during** (TRAUMATIC EVENT)? **Since** (TRAUMATIC EVENT), **how long has this gone on? (Almost all of the time for more than 1 month?)**

IF LIFETIME RATING OF "+": **Has this also happened in the past month, since** (ONE MONTH AGO)? **Has it been almost all of the time during the past month?**

1. Avoidance of, or efforts to avoid distressing memories, thoughts, or feelings about or closely associated with the traumatic event(s).

—　　+

Past month
—　　+

G20

G21

...**have there been things, places, or people that you have tried to avoid because it brought up upsetting memories, thoughts, or feelings about** (TRAUMATIC EVENT)? **How long has this gone on? (Almost all of the time for more than 1 month?)**

   IF NO: **How about avoiding certain activities, situations, or topics of conversation? Since** (TRAUMATIC EVENT), **how long has this gone on? (Almost all of the time for more than 1 month?)**

IF LIFETIME RATING OF "+": **Has this also happened in the past month? Has it been almost all of the time during the past month?**

2. Avoidance of or efforts to avoid external reminders (people, places, conversations, activities, objects, situations), that arouse distressing memories, thoughts, or feelings about or closely associated with the traumatic event(s).

—　　+

Past month
—　　+

G21

G22

AT LEAST ONE OF THE ABOVE CRITERION C SXS **(G20–G21)** IS RATED "+".

NO　　YES

If other reported traumatic events, consider returning to **G13** and reassessing PTSD for that event. Otherwise, go to **H1** (ADHD), **page 86**.

Criterion C met past month.

NO　　YES

G22

	Since (TRAUMATIC EVENT)…	D. Negative alterations in cognitions and mood associated with the traumatic event(s), beginning or worsening after the traumatic event(s) occurred, as evidenced by two (or more) of the following:		
G23	…have you been unable to remember some important part of what happened? (Tell me about that.) IF YES: **Did you get a head injury during (TRAUMATIC EVENT)? Were you drinking a lot or were taking any drugs at the time of (TRAUMATIC EVENT)?** IF LIFETIME RATING OF "+": **Has this also been the case in the past month, since (ONE MONTH AGO)? How many times?**	1. Inability to remember an important aspect of the traumatic event(s) (typically due to dissociative amnesia and not to other factors such as head injury, alcohol, or drugs).	— + ↓ Past month — +	G23
G24	……has there been a change in how you think about yourself? (Like feeling you are "bad," or permanently damaged or "broken"?) Tell me about that. How long have you felt this way about yourself? (Have you felt this way almost all of the time for more than 1 month?) IF NO: **Has there been a change in how you see other people or the way the world works? Like you can't trust anyone anymore? Like the world is a completely dangerous place? Tell me about that. How long have you thought this way? (Have you thought this way almost all of the time for more than 1 month?)** IF LIFETIME RATING OF "+": **Has this also been the case in the past month? How much of the time? (Almost all of the time?)**	2. Persistent and exaggerated negative beliefs or expectations about oneself, others, or the world (e.g., "I am bad," "No one can be trusted," "The world is completely dangerous," "My whole nervous system is permanently ruined").	— + ↓ Past month — +	G24
G25	…have you blamed yourself for the (TRAUMATIC EVENT) or how it affected your life? (Like thinking that [TRAUMATIC EVENT] was your fault or that you should have done something to prevent it? Like thinking that you should have gotten over it by now?) → IF YES: **Tell me about it. How long have you thought this way? (Have you thought this way almost all of the time for more than 1 month?)** → IF NO: **Have you blamed someone else for (TRAUMATIC EVENT)? Tell me about that. (What did they have to do with [TRAUMATIC EVENT]?) How long have you thought it was their fault? (Have you thought this way almost all of the time for more than 1 month?)** IF LIFETIME RATING OF "+": **Has this also been the case in the past month? How much of the time? (Almost all of the time?)**	3. Persistent, distorted cognitions about the cause or consequences of the traumatic event(s) that lead the individual to blame himself/herself or others.	— + ↓ Past month — +	G25

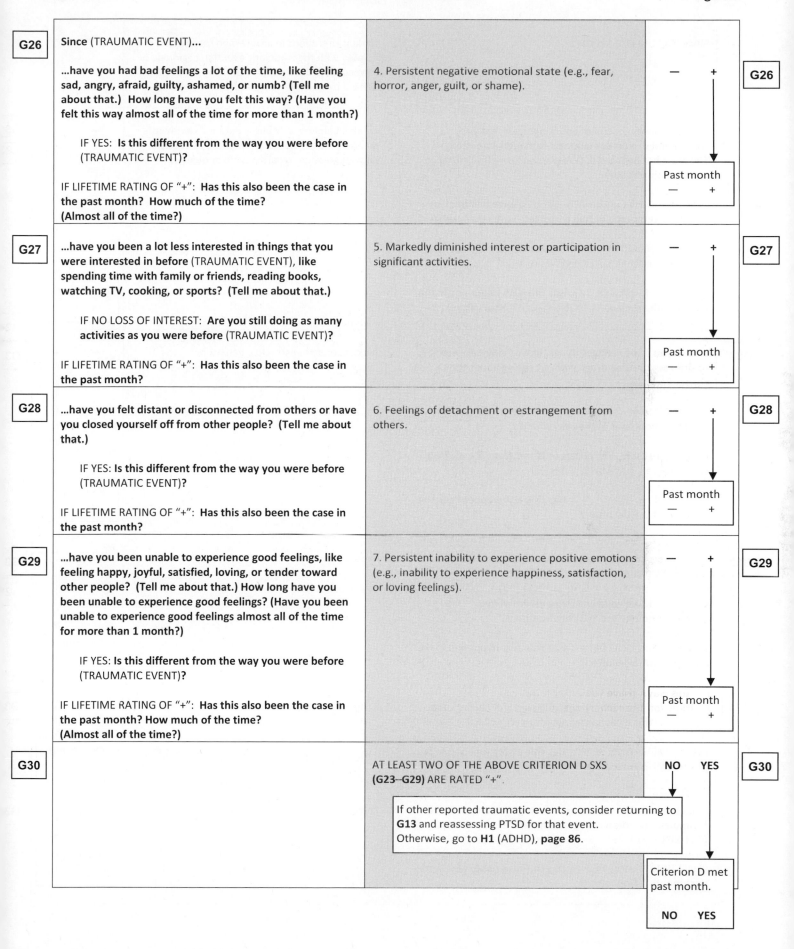

G26 | Since (TRAUMATIC EVENT)...

...have you had bad feelings a lot of the time, like feeling sad, angry, afraid, guilty, ashamed, or numb? (Tell me about that.) How long have you felt this way? (Have you felt this way almost all of the time for more than 1 month?)

    IF YES: **Is this different from the way you were before (TRAUMATIC EVENT)?**

IF LIFETIME RATING OF "+": **Has this also been the case in the past month? How much of the time? (Almost all of the time?)**

| 4. Persistent negative emotional state (e.g., fear, horror, anger, guilt, or shame). | −   +

 Past month
   −   + | **G26** |

G27 | ...have you been a lot less interested in things that you were interested in before (TRAUMATIC EVENT), like spending time with family or friends, reading books, watching TV, cooking, or sports? (Tell me about that.)

    IF NO LOSS OF INTEREST: **Are you still doing as many activities as you were before (TRAUMATIC EVENT)?**

IF LIFETIME RATING OF "+": **Has this also been the case in the past month?**

| 5. Markedly diminished interest or participation in significant activities. | −   +

 Past month
   −   + | **G27** |

G28 | ...have you felt distant or disconnected from others or have you closed yourself off from other people? (Tell me about that.)

    IF YES: **Is this different from the way you were before (TRAUMATIC EVENT)?**

IF LIFETIME RATING OF "+": **Has this also been the case in the past month?**

| 6. Feelings of detachment or estrangement from others. | −   +

 Past month
   −   + | **G28** |

G29 | ...have you been unable to experience good feelings, like feeling happy, joyful, satisfied, loving, or tender toward other people? (Tell me about that.) How long have you been unable to experience good feelings? (Have you been unable to experience good feelings almost all of the time for more than 1 month?)

    IF YES: **Is this different from the way you were before (TRAUMATIC EVENT)?**

IF LIFETIME RATING OF "+": **Has this also been the case in the past month? How much of the time? (Almost all of the time?)**

| 7. Persistent inability to experience positive emotions (e.g., inability to experience happiness, satisfaction, or loving feelings). | −   +

 Past month
   −   + | **G29** |

G30 | | AT LEAST TWO OF THE ABOVE CRITERION D SXS (**G23–G29**) ARE RATED "+".

NO   YES

If other reported traumatic events, consider returning to **G13** and reassessing PTSD for that event. Otherwise, go to **H1** (ADHD), **page 86**.

Criterion D met past month.

NO   YES | **G30** |

	Since (TRAUMATIC EVENT)...	E. Marked alterations in arousal and reactivity associated with the traumatic event(s), beginning or worsening after the traumatic event(s) occurred, as evidenced by two (or more) of the following:		
G31	...have you lost control of your anger, so that you threatened or hurt someone or damaged something? Tell me what happened. (Was it over something little or even nothing at all?) IF NO: **Since** (TRAUMATIC EVENT), **have you been more quick-tempered or had a shorter "fuse" than before?** IF YES TO EITHER: **How different is this from the way you were before** (TRAUMATIC EVENT)? IF LIFETIME RATING OF "+": **Has this also happened in the past month, since** (ONE MONTH AGO)? **How often?**	1. Irritable behavior and angry outbursts (with little or no provocation) typically expressed as verbal or physical aggression toward people or objects.	— + Past month — +	**G3**
G32	...have you done reckless things, like driving dangerously, or drinking or using drugs without caring about the consequences? IF NO: **How about hurting yourself on purpose or trying to kill yourself?** (What did you do?) IF YES TO ETIHER: **How different is this from the way you were before** (TRAUMATIC EVENT)? IF LIFETIME RATING OF "+": **Has this also happened in the past month? How often?**	2. Reckless or self-destructive behavior.	— + Past month — +	**G3**
G33	...have you noticed that you have been more watchful or on guard? (What are some examples?) IF NO: **Have you been extra aware of your surroundings and your environment?** IF LIFETIME RATING OF "+": **Has this also happened in the past month? How often?**	3. Hypervigilance.	— + Past month — +	**G3**
G34	...have you been jumpy or easily startled, like by sudden noises? (Is this a change from before [TRAUMATIC EVENT]?) IF LIFETIME RATING OF "+": **Has this also happened in the past month? How often?**	4. Exaggerated startle response.	— + Past month — +	**G3**
G35	...have you had trouble concentrating? (What are some examples? (Is this a change from before [TRAUMATIC EVENT]?) IF LIFETIME RATING OF "+": **Has this also happened in the past month? How often?**	5. Problems with concentration.	— + Past month — +	**G3**

G36	**Since** (TRAUMATIC EVENT)... **...how have you been sleeping since (TRAUMATIC EVENT)? (Is this a change from before [TRAUMATIC EVENT]?)** IF LIFETIME RATING OF "+": **Has this also happened in the past month? How often?**	6. Sleep disturbance (e.g., difficulty falling or staying asleep or restless sleep).	— + ↓ Past month — +	**G36**

G37

AT LEAST TWO OF THE ABOVE CRITERION E SXS **(G31–G36)** ARE RATED "+".

NO   YES

If other reported traumatic events, consider returning to **G13** and reassessing PTSD for that event.
Otherwise, go to **H1** (ADHD), **page 86**.

Criterion E met past month.

NO   YES

G38 | **About how long did these** (PTSD SXS RATED "+") **last altogether?**

F. Duration of the disturbance [symptoms in Criteria B **(G19)**, C **(G22)**, D **(G30)**, and E **(G37)**] is more than 1 month.

— +   **G38**

If other reported traumatic events, consider returning to **G13** and reassessing PTSD for that event.
Otherwise, go to **H1** (ADHD), **page 86**.

G39 | IF UNCLEAR: **What effect did** (PTSD SXS) **have on your life?**

ASK THE FOLLOWING QUESTIONS <u>ONLY AS NEEDED</u>:

How have (PTSD SXS) **affected your relationships or your interactions with other people? (Have [PTSD SXS] caused you any problems in your relationships with your family, romantic partner, or friends?)**

How have (PTSD SXS) **affected your work/school? (How about your attendance at work/school? Have [PTSD SXS] made it more difficult to do your work/schoolwork? Have [PTSD SXS] affected the quality of your work/schoolwork?)**

How have [PTSD SXS] **affected your ability to take care of things at home? What about being involved in things that are important to you, like religious activities, physical exercise, or hobbies?**

Have (PTSD SXS) **affected any other important part of your life?**

IF HAVE NOT INTERFERED WITH LIFE: **How much have you been bothered or upset by** (PTSD SXS)?

IF LIFETIME RATING OF "+": **How have** (PTSD SXS) **affected your life in the past month?**

G. The disturbance causes clinically significant distress or impairment in social, occupational, or other important areas of functioning.

— +   **G39**

If other reported traumatic events, consider returning to **G13** and reassessing PTSD for that event.
Otherwise, go to **H1** (ADHD), **page 86**.

Past month
— +

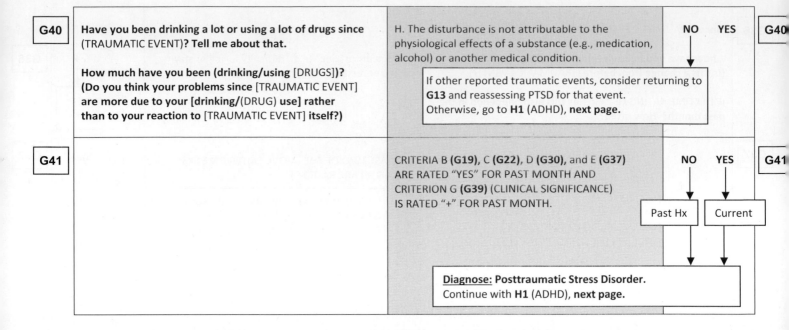

G40   **Have you been drinking a lot or using a lot of drugs since (TRAUMATIC EVENT)? Tell me about that.**

How much have you been (drinking/using [DRUGS])? (Do you think your problems since [TRAUMATIC EVENT] are more due to your [drinking/(DRUG) use] rather than to your reaction to [TRAUMATIC EVENT] itself?)

H. The disturbance is not attributable to the physiological effects of a substance (e.g., medication, alcohol) or another medical condition.   NO   YES   **G40**

If other reported traumatic events, consider returning to **G13** and reassessing PTSD for that event. Otherwise, go to **H1** (ADHD), **next page.**

G41   CRITERIA B **(G19)**, C **(G22)**, D **(G30)**, and E **(G37)** ARE RATED "YES" FOR PAST MONTH AND CRITERION G **(G39)** (CLINICAL SIGNIFICANCE) IS RATED "+" FOR PAST MONTH.   NO   YES   **G41**

Past Hx   Current

**Diagnose: Posttraumatic Stress Disorder.** Continue with **H1** (ADHD), **next page.**

H. ADULT ATTENTION-DEFICIT/HYPERACTIVITY DISORDER

	CURRENT ATTENTION-DEFICIT/HYPERACTIVITY DISORDER (PAST 6 MONTHS, ADULTS)	ATTENTION-DEFICIT/HYPERACTIVITY DISORDER CRITERIA		
H1	Over the past several years, have you been easily distracted or disorganized? IF NO: **Over the past several years, have you had a lot of difficulty sitting still or waiting your turn?** IF THERE IS NO EVIDENCE THAT THE PERSON HAS BEEN DISTRACTED, DISORGANIZED, IMPULSIVE, OR UNABLE TO SIT STILL OVER THE PAST 6 MONTHS, CHECK HERE ___ AND GO TO I1 (Screening), **page 91.**	A. A persistent pattern of inattention and/or hyperactivity-impulsivity that interferes with functioning or development, as characterized by (1) and/or (2):	**H1**	
	Thinking about how you have been over the past 6 months, since (6 MONTHS AGO)…	1. **Inattention:** Five (or more) of the following symptoms have persisted for at least 6 months to a degree that is inconsistent with developmental level and that negatively impacts directly on social and academic/occupational activities: **Note:** The symptoms are not solely a manifestation of oppositional behavior, defiance, hostility, or failure to understand tasks or instructions.		
H2	…have you often missed important details or made mistakes at work (or school) or while taking care of things at home? Please give me some examples. (Have you often made mistakes balancing your checkbook or paying bills? Have other people complained that you don't pay enough attention to detail or that your work is careless?)	a. Often fails to give close attention to details or makes careless mistakes in schoolwork, at work, or during other activities (e.g., overlooks or misses details, work is inaccurate).	− +	**H2**
H3	…have you often had trouble staying focused on things like reading a book, following a conversation, or doing household chores? Give me some examples.	b. Often has difficulty sustaining attention in tasks or play activities (e.g., has difficulty remaining focused during lectures, conversations, or lengthy reading).	− +	**H3**
H4	…has anyone commented or complained that you haven't seemed to be listening or that your mind was elsewhere while they were talking? Tell me about that. (How often has this happened?) (Has this happened even when nothing else is going on…when there are no obvious distractions?)	c. Often does not seem to listen when spoken to directly (e.g., mind seems elsewhere, even in the absence of any obvious distraction).	− +	**H4**
H5	…have you often started things and then dropped them without finishing because you lost your focus or got sidetracked? Give me some examples.	d. Often does not follow through on instructions and fails to finish schoolwork, chores, or duties in the workplace (e.g., starts tasks but quickly loses focus and is easily sidetracked).	− +	**H5**

H6	**In the past 6 months, since** (SIX MONTHS AGO)... **...have you had trouble organizing things at home or at work, or staying on top of things? Tell me about that. (Are your desk and closet so messy and disorganized that you have had trouble finding things? Have you had trouble managing your time so that you have been late a lot or missed appointments or failed to meet deadlines?)**	e. Often has difficulty organizing tasks and activities (e.g., difficulty managing sequential tasks; difficulty keeping materials and belongings in order; messy, disorganized work; has poor time management; fails to meet deadlines).	–	+	H
H7	**...have you typically avoided or strongly disliked tasks or jobs that require concentrating on details for extended periods, things like preparing a report for work or writing a paper? Give me some examples of the types of tasks or jobs you have avoided or disliked.**	f. Often avoids, dislikes, or is reluctant to engage in tasks that require sustained mental effort (e.g., schoolwork or homework, for older adolescents and adults, preparing reports, completing forms, reviewing lengthy papers).	–	+	H
H8	**...have you often lost or misplaced things like your wallet, your glasses, your keys, or your cell phone? How about files at work or tools you needed for work? Tell me about that.**	g. Often loses things necessary for tasks or activities (e.g., school materials, pencils, books, tools, wallets, keys, paperwork, eyeglasses, mobile telephones).	–	+	H
H9	**...have you been very easily distracted by things going on around you that most others would have easily ignored, like a car honking or other people talking? Tell me about that.** IF NO: **Have you often gotten distracted by your own thoughts that were unrelated to what you were doing?**	h. Is often easily distracted by extraneous stimuli (for older adolescents and adults, may include unrelated thoughts).	–	+	H
H10	**...have you often been very forgetful, for example, forgetting to return phone calls, forgetting to pay bills, or forgetting appointments? Tell me about that.**	i. Is often forgetful in everyday activities (e.g., doing chores, running errands; for older adolescents and adults, returning calls, paying bills, keeping appointments).	–	+	H1
H11		AT LEAST FIVE OF THE ABOVE CRITERION A1 (INATTENTION) SXS **(H2–H10)** ARE RATED "+".	NO	YES ↓ ADHD Criterion A1 is met.	H1

	Thinking about how you have been over the past 6 months, since (6 MONTHS AGO)...	2. **Hyperactivity and impulsivity**: Five (or more) of the following symptoms have persisted for at least 6 months to a degree that is inconsistent with developmental level and that negatively impacts directly on social and academic/occupational activities: **Note:** The symptoms are not solely a manifestation of oppositional behavior, defiance, hostility, or a failure to understand tasks or instructions.			
H12	...have you often fidgeted or squirmed or tapped your foot when you were in a situation where you have had to sit still, like on a plane, in class, or at meetings? Tell me about that.	a. Often fidgets with or taps hands or feet or squirms in seat.	—	+	**H12**
H13	...have you often left your seat when you were expected to stay seated, for example, during a religious service, in a movie theater, in class, or at meetings? Tell me about that.	b. Often leaves seat in situations when remaining seated is expected (e.g., leaves his or her place in the classroom, in the office or other workplace, or in other situations that require remaining in place).	—	+	**H13**
H14	...have you often felt physically restless, especially when you had to stay put for a while? Tell me about that.	c. Often runs about or climbs in situations where it is inappropriate. (**Note:** In adolescents or adults, may be limited to feeling restless.)	—	+	**H14**
H15	...have you often been unable to do something quietly in your spare time, like reading a book? Tell me about that. (Have others said that you talk too much or that you make too much noise when you are supposed to be quiet?)	d. Often unable to play or engage in leisure activities quietly.	—	+	**H15**
H16	...have you often felt like you always have to be moving or doing something? Have you been uncomfortable being still for any length of time? Have others told you that you are hard to keep up with? Have other people told you that being with you is exhausting or draining? Tell me about that.	e. Is often "on the go," acting as if "driven by a motor" (e.g., is unable to be or uncomfortable being still for extended time, as in restaurants, meetings; may be experienced by others as being restless or difficult to keep up with).	—	+	**H16**
H17	...have you often talked too much? Tell me about that. (Have other people complained that you talk too much? How often does this happen?)	f. Often talks excessively.	—	+	**H17**
H18	...have you often finished people's sentences or blurted out an answer before the other person finished asking the question? Tell me about that. (Has it often been hard for you to wait your turn in conversations?)	g. Often blurts out an answer before a question has been completed (e.g., completes people's sentences; cannot wait for turn in conversation.	—	+	**H18**
H19	...have you often had trouble waiting for your "turn," like while waiting in line or ordering at a restaurant? Describe what happens.	h. Often has difficulty waiting his or her turn (e.g., while waiting in line).	—	+	**H19**

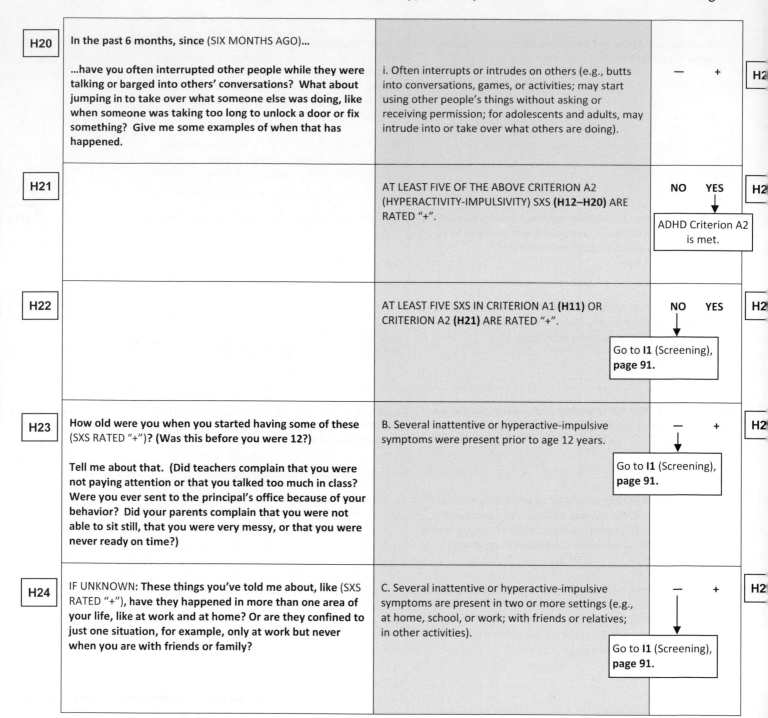

H20

In the past 6 months, since (SIX MONTHS AGO)...

...have you often interrupted other people while they were talking or barged into others' conversations? What about jumping in to take over what someone else was doing, like when someone was taking too long to unlock a door or fix something? Give me some examples of when that has happened.

i. Often interrupts or intrudes on others (e.g., butts into conversations, games, or activities; may start using other people's things without asking or receiving permission; for adolescents and adults, may intrude into or take over what others are doing).

—   +   **H2**

H21

AT LEAST FIVE OF THE ABOVE CRITERION A2 (HYPERACTIVITY-IMPULSIVITY) SXS **(H12–H20)** ARE RATED "+".

NO   YES   **H2**

ADHD Criterion A2 is met.

H22

AT LEAST FIVE SXS IN CRITERION A1 **(H11)** OR CRITERION A2 **(H21)** ARE RATED "+".

NO   YES   **H2**

Go to **I1** (Screening), **page 91.**

H23

How old were you when you started having some of these (SXS RATED "+")? **(Was this before you were 12?)**

Tell me about that. **(Did teachers complain that you were not paying attention or that you talked too much in class? Were you ever sent to the principal's office because of your behavior? Did your parents complain that you were not able to sit still, that you were very messy, or that you were never ready on time?)**

B. Several inattentive or hyperactive-impulsive symptoms were present prior to age 12 years.

—   +   **H2**

Go to **I1** (Screening), **page 91.**

H24

IF UNKNOWN: **These things you've told me about, like** (SXS RATED "+"), **have they happened in more than one area of your life, like at work and at home? Or are they confined to just one situation, for example, only at work but never when you are with friends or family?**

C. Several inattentive or hyperactive-impulsive symptoms are present in two or more settings (e.g., at home, school, or work; with friends or relatives; in other activities).

—   +   **H2**

Go to **I1** (Screening), **page 91.**

H25

IF UNCLEAR: **What effect have** (ADHD SXS) **had on your life in the past 6 months, since** (6 MONTHS AGO)?

ASK THE FOLLOWING QUESTIONS <u>ONLY AS NEEDED</u>:

How have (ADHD SXS) **affected your relationships or your interactions with other people? (Have** [ADHD SXS] **caused you any problems in your relationships with your family, romantic partner, or friends?)**

How have (ADHD SXS) **affected your work/school? (How about your attendance at work/school? Have** [ADHD SXS] **made it more difficult to do your work/schoolwork? Have** [ADHD SXS] **affected the quality of your work/schoolwork?)**

How have (ADHD SXS) **affected your ability to take care of things at home? Have your** (ADHD SXS) **made it hard for you to do things that are important to you, like religious activities, physical exercise, sports, or hobbies?**

Have (ADHD SXS) **affected any other important part of your life?**

D. There is clear evidence that the symptoms interfere with, or reduce the quality of, social, academic, or occupational functioning.

     −   +

Go to **I1** (Screening), **next page.**

H25

H26

IF A PSYCHOTIC DISORDER HAS BEEN DIAGNOSED: **Did you have** (ADHD SXS RATED "+") **before you had** (SXS OF PSYCHOTIC DISORDER)?

E. The symptoms do not occur exclusively during the course of Schizophrenia or another Psychotic Disorder and are not better explained by another mental disorder (e.g., Depressive Disorder, Bipolar Disorder, Anxiety Disorder, Dissociative Disorder, Personality Disorder, Substance Intoxication or Withdrawal).

NO   **YES**

Go to **I1** (Screening), **next page.**

H26

Diagnose: Attention-Deficit/Hyperactivity Disorder (current)
Combined Presentation: If Criterion A1/item **H11, page 87** (inattention) and Criterion A2/item **H21, page 89** (hyperactivity-impulsivity) are met for the past 6 months.
Predominantly Inattentive Presentation: If Criterion A1/item **H11, page 87** (inattention) is met but Criterion A2/item **H21, page 89** (hyperactivity-impulsivity) is not met for the past 6 months.
Predominantly Hyperactive/Impulsive Presentation: If Criterion A2/item **H21, page 89** (hyperactivity-impulsivity) is met but Criterion A1/item **H11, page 87** (inattention) is not met for the past 6 months.

Go to **I1** (Screening), **next page.**

I. SCREENING FOR OTHER CURRENT DISORDERS

Now I'm going to ask you just a few more questions about other problems you may be experiencing.

IF THE ANSWER TO ANY OF THE FOLLOWING QUESTIONS IS "YES," FOLLOW UP WITH ADDITIONAL QUESTIONS, SUCH AS, "**Tell me more about that,**" "**Is this causing a problem for you or interfering with your life?**" AND "**Are you currently getting help for that?**"

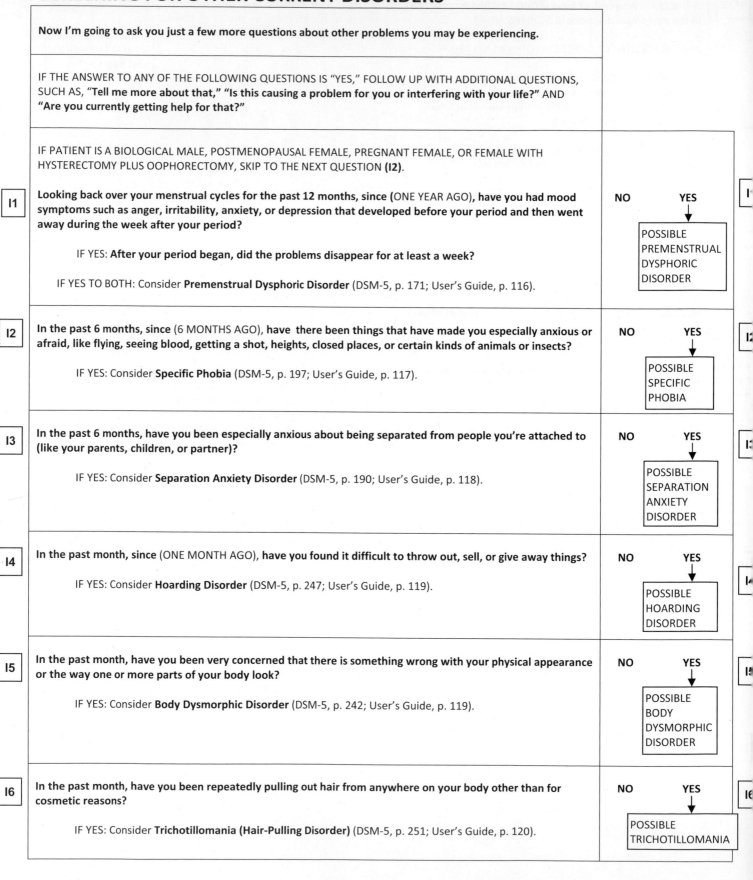

I1

IF PATIENT IS A BIOLOGICAL MALE, POSTMENOPAUSAL FEMALE, PREGNANT FEMALE, OR FEMALE WITH HYSTERECTOMY PLUS OOPHORECTOMY, SKIP TO THE NEXT QUESTION **(I2)**.

Looking back over your menstrual cycles for the past 12 months, since (ONE YEAR AGO), **have you had mood symptoms such as anger, irritability, anxiety, or depression that developed before your period and then went away during the week after your period?**

    IF YES: **After your period began, did the problems disappear for at least a week?**

    IF YES TO BOTH: Consider **Premenstrual Dysphoric Disorder** (DSM-5, p. 171; User's Guide, p. 116).

NO   YES

POSSIBLE PREMENSTRUAL DYSPHORIC DISORDER

I2

In the past 6 months, since (6 MONTHS AGO), **have there been things that have made you especially anxious or afraid, like flying, seeing blood, getting a shot, heights, closed places, or certain kinds of animals or insects?**

    IF YES: Consider **Specific Phobia** (DSM-5, p. 197; User's Guide, p. 117).

NO   YES

POSSIBLE SPECIFIC PHOBIA

I3

In the past 6 months, have you been especially anxious about being separated from people you're attached to (like your parents, children, or partner)?

    IF YES: Consider **Separation Anxiety Disorder** (DSM-5, p. 190; User's Guide, p. 118).

NO   YES

POSSIBLE SEPARATION ANXIETY DISORDER

I4

In the past month, since (ONE MONTH AGO), **have you found it difficult to throw out, sell, or give away things?**

    IF YES: Consider **Hoarding Disorder** (DSM-5, p. 247; User's Guide, p. 119).

NO   YES

POSSIBLE HOARDING DISORDER

I5

In the past month, have you been very concerned that there is something wrong with your physical appearance or the way one or more parts of your body look?

    IF YES: Consider **Body Dysmorphic Disorder** (DSM-5, p. 242; User's Guide, p. 119).

NO   YES

POSSIBLE BODY DYSMORPHIC DISORDER

I6

In the past month, have you been repeatedly pulling out hair from anywhere on your body other than for cosmetic reasons?

    IF YES: Consider **Trichotillomania (Hair-Pulling Disorder)** (DSM-5, p. 251; User's Guide, p. 120).

NO   YES

POSSIBLE TRICHOTILLOMANIA

I7	In the past month, have you been repeatedly picking at your skin with your fingernails, tweezers, pins, or other objects? IF YES: Consider **Excoriation (Skin-Picking) Disorder** (DSM-5, p. 254; User's Guide, p. 120).	NO YES POSSIBLE EXCORIATION DISORDER	**I7**
I8	Over the past 3 months, since (3 MONTHS AGO), **has a major concern of yours been that you are not getting enough good sleep or not feeling rested?** IF YES: Consider **Insomnia Disorder** (DSM-5, p. 362; User's Guide, p. 121).	NO YES POSSIBLE INSOMNIA DISORDER	**I8**
I9	Over the past 3 months, have you often had days when you were sleepy despite having slept for at least 7 hours? IF YES: Consider **Hypersomnolence Disorder** (DSM-5, p. 368; User's Guide, p. 121).	NO YES POSSIBLE HYPERSOMNOLENCE DISORDER	**I9**
I10	In the past 3 months, have you had a time when you weighed much less than other people thought you ought to weigh? IF YES: Consider **Anorexia Nervosa** (DSM-5, p. 338; User's Guide, p. 122).	NO YES POSSIBLE ANOREXIA NERVOSA	**I10**
I11	In the past 3 months, have you had eating binges, that is, times when you couldn't resist eating a lot of food or stop eating once you started? IF YES: Consider **Bulimia Nervosa** (DSM-5, p. 345; User's Guide, p. 122) or **Binge-Eating Disorder** (DSM-5, p. 350; User's Guide, p. 123).	NO YES POSSIBLE BULIMIA NERVOSA OR BINGE-EATING DISORDER	**I11**
I12	In the past month, since (ONE MONTH AGO), **have you been uninterested in food in general or have you kept forgetting to eat?** IF NO: **In the past month, have you avoided eating a lot of foods because of the way they look or the way they feel in your mouth?** IF NO: **In the past month, have you avoided eating a lot of different foods because you are afraid you won't be able to swallow or that you will choke, gag, or throw up?** IF YES TO ANY: Consider **Avoidant/Restrictive Food Intake Disorder** (DSM-5, p. 334; User's Guide, p. 123).	NO YES POSSIBLE AVOIDANT/ RESTRICTIVE FOOD INTAKE DISORDER	**I12**
I13	Over the past 6 months, since (6 MONTHS AGO), **have you been bothered by any physical symptoms?** IF YES: Consider **Somatic Symptom Disorder** (DSM-5, p. 311; User's Guide, p. 124).	NO YES POSSIBLE SOMATIC SYMPTOM DISORDER	**I13**

I14	Over the past 6 months, have you spent a lot of time thinking that you have, or will get, a serious disease?
	
	    IF YES: Consider **Illness Anxiety Disorder** (DSM-5, p. 315; User's Guide, p. 124).
		NO YES
		      ↓
		POSSIBLE ILLNESS ANXIETY DISORDER
			I14

I15	In the past 12 months, since (ONE YEAR AGO), **have you had periods in which you frequently lost control of your temper and ended up yelling or getting into arguments with others?**
	
	    IF NO: **In the past year, have you lost your temper so that you shoved, hit, kicked, or threw something at a person or an animal or damaged someone's property?**
	
	  IF YES TO EITHER: Consider **Intermittent Explosive Disorder** (DSM-5, p. 466; User's Guide, p. 125).
		NO YES
		      ↓
		POSSIBLE INTERMITTENT EXPLOSIVE DISORDER
			I15

I16	In the past 12 months, **have you regularly gambled or regularly bought lottery tickets?**
	
	    IF YES: Consider **Gambling Disorder** (DSM-5, p. 585; User's Guide, p. 126).
		NO YES
		      ↓
		POSSIBLE GAMBLING DISORDER
			I16

Go to **J1**, (Adjustment Disorder), **next page.**

J. ADJUSTMENT DISORDER

CURRENT ADJUSTMENT DISORDER (PAST 6 MONTHS)	ADJUSTMENT DISORDER CRITERIA	

CONSIDER ADJUSTMENT DISORDER ONLY IF 1) THERE IS AN IDENTIFIED STRESSOR AND 2) THERE ARE SYMPTOMS OCCURRING IN THE PAST 6 MONTHS THAT DO NOT MEET THE CRITERIA FOR ANOTHER DSM-5 DISORDER.

IF SYMPTOMS MEET CRITERIA FOR A DSM-5 DISORDER <u>NOT</u> INCLUDED IN THE SCID-5-CV, OR MEET THE DEFINITIONAL REQUIREMENTS FOR AN OTHER OR UNSPECIFIED CATEGORY NOT INCLUDED IN THE SCID-5-CV (E.G., OTHER SPECIFIED OR UNSPECIFIED ANXIETY DISORDER), RECORD THAT DISORDER AND THE ICD-10-CM DIAGNOSTIC CODE AT THE BOTTOM OF PAGE 4 OF THE DIAGNOSTIC SUMMARY SCORE SHEET.

OTHERWISE THE SCID-5-CV HAS BEEEN COMPLETED.

J1

INFORMATION OBTAINED FROM OVERVIEW OF PRESENT ILLNESS WILL USUALLY BE SUFFICIENT TO RATE THIS CRITERION.

IF UNKNOWN: **Did anything happen to you before** (SXS) **began?**

    IF YES: **Tell me about what happened. Do you think that** (STRESSOR) **had anything to do with your developing** (SXS)**?**

    ▶ IF SINGLE EVENT: **How long after** (STRESSOR) **did you first develop** (SXS)**? (Was it within 3 months?)**

    ▶ IF CHRONIC STRESSOR: **How long after** (STRESSOR) **began did you first develop** (SXS)**? (Was it within 3 months?)**

A. The development of emotional or behavioral symptoms in response to an identifiable stressor(s) occurring within 3 months of the onset of the stressor(s).

− +
↓
END OF SCID-5-CV

J1

J2

IF UNKNOWN: **What effect did** (SXS) **have on your life?**

ASK THE FOLLOWING QUESTIONS <u>AS NEEDED</u>:

How have (SXS) **affected your relationships or your interactions with other people? (Have [SXS] caused you any problems in your relationships with your family, romantic partner, or friends?)**

How have (SXS) **affected your work/school? (How about your attendance at work/school? Have [SXS] made it more difficult to do your work/schoolwork? Have [SXS] affected the quality of your work/schoolwork?)**

How have (SXS) **affected your ability to take care of things at home? What about being involved in things that are important to you, like religious activities, physical exercise, or hobbies?**

Have (SXS) **affected any other important part of your life?**

IF DO NOT INTERFERE WITH LIFE: **How much have you been bothered or upset by having** (SXS)**?**

B. These symptoms or behaviors are clinically significant, as evidenced by one or both of the following:

1. Marked distress that is out of proportion to the severity or intensity of the stressor, taking into account the external context and the cultural factors that might influence symptom severity and presentation.

2. Significant impairment in social, occupational, or other important areas of functioning.

− +
↓
END OF SCID-5-CV

J2

J3	(Have you had this kind of reaction many times before?) (Were you having these [SXS] **even before** [STRESSOR] **happened?**)	C. The stress-related disturbance does not meet the criteria for another mental disorder and is not merely an exacerbation of a preexisting mental disorder [including Personality Disorder].	NO YES ↓ END OF SCID-5-CV	J
J4	IF UNKNOWN: **Did someone close to you die just before** (SXS)**?**	D. The symptoms do not represent normal bereavement.	NO YES ↓ END OF SCID-5-CV	J
J5	IF UNKNOWN: **How long has it been since** (STRESSOR AND ITS CONSEQUENCES) **was over?**	E. Once the stressor or its consequences have terminated, the symptoms do not persist for more than an additional 6 months.	— + ↓ END OF SCID-5-CV	J

Diagnose: **Adjustment Disorder (current)**
With Depressed Mood: Low mood, tearfulness, or feelings of hopelessness are predominant.
With Anxiety: Nervousness, worry, jitteriness, or separation anxiety is predominant.
With Mixed Anxiety and Depressed Mood: A combination of depression and anxiety is predominant.
With Disturbance of Conduct: Disturbance of conduct is predominant.
With Mixed Disturbance of Emotions and Conduct: Both emotional symptoms (e.g., depression, anxiety) and a disturbance of conduct are predominant.
Unspecified: For maladaptive reactions that are not classifiable as one of the specific subtypes of Adjustment Disorder.